A Case-Based Approach

to Emergency Psychiatry

A Case-Based Approach to Emergency Psychiatry

EDITED BY KATHERINE MALOY, MD

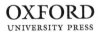

OXFORD
UNIVERSITY PRESS

Oxford University Press is a department of the University of Oxford. It furthers
the University's objective of excellence in research, scholarship, and education
by publishing worldwide. Oxford is a registered trade mark of Oxford University
Press in the UK and certain other countries.

Published in the United States of America by Oxford University Press
198 Madison Avenue, New York, NY 10016, United States of America.

Cataloging-in-Publication data is on file at the Library of Congress
ISBN 978-0-19-025084-3

9 8 7 6 5 4 3 2

Printed by Webcom, Inc., Canada

CONTENTS

Adria N. Adams, PsyD
Clinical Director
Interim Crisis Clinic
Bellevue Hospital
Comprehensive Psychiatric
    Emergency Department
NYU Clinical Faculty
New York University
New York, NY

Luke Archibald, MD
Clinical Assistant Professor
New York University School of
    Medicine
Unit Chief
Bellevue Hospital 20 East Dual
    Diagnosis
New York University School
    of Medicine
New York, NY

Bem Atim, MD
Psychaitry Resident
New York University School
    of Medicine
New York, NY

Wiktoria Bielska, MD
Assistant Clinical Professor
New York University School
    of Medicine
Attending Psychiatrist
Bellevue Hospital Comprehensive
    Psychiatric Emergency Program
New York, NY

Gillian Copeland, MD, MBA
Chief Resident, Department
    of Psychiatry
New York University
New York, NY

Abigail L. Dahan, MD, FAPA
Attending Psychiatrist
Bellevue Comprehensive Psychiatric
    Emergency Program
Clinical Assistant Professor
Department of Psychiatry
New York University School
    of Medicine
New York, NY

Anthony Dark, MD
Attending Psychiatrist
Comprehensive Psychiatric Emergency
    Program
Bellevue Hospital Center
Clinical Assistant Professor
New York University School
    of Medicine
New York, NY

Emily Deringer, MD
Clinical Assistant Professor
Department of Psychiatry
New York University School
    of Medicine
Attending Psychiatrist
Bellevue Comprehensive Psychiatric
    Emergency Program
New York, NY

Ruth S. Gerson, MD
Director, Bellevue Hospital Children's
  Comprehensive Psychiatric
  Emergency Program
Clinical Assistant Professor
Department of Child and Adolescent
  Psychiatry
New York University School
  of Medicine
New York, NY

Jennifer Goldman, MD
Attending Psychiatrist
Bellevue Medical Center
Comprehensive Psychiatric
  Emergency Program
Clinical Assistant Professor
Department of Psychiatry
New York University Medical Center
New York, NY

Lindsay Gurin, MD
Resident, Combined Psychiatry/
  Neurology Program
Departments of Psychiatry and
  Neurology
New York University School
  of Medicine
New York, NY

Fadi Haddad, MD
Director of Child Psychiatric
  Emergency Services
Bellevue Hospital Center
Clinical Assistant Professor
Department of Child and
  Adolescent Psychiatry
New York University School
  of Medicine
New York, NY

Jonathan Howard, MD
Assistant Professor of Neurology
  and Psychiatry
New York University
New York, NY

Joe Kwon, MD
Attending Psychiatrist
Bellevue Hospital Center
Assistant Clinical Professor
New York University Department
  of Psychiatry
New York, NY

Rebecca Lewis, MD
Attending Psychiatrist
Bellevue Comprehensive Psychiatric
  Emergency Program
Clinical Assistant Professor
  of Psychiatry
New York University School
  of Medicine
New York, NY

Camilla Lyons, MD, MPH
Attending Psychiatrist
Bellevue Comprehensive Psychiatric
  Emergency Program
Clinical Assistant Professor
Department of Psychiatry
New York University School
  of Medicine
New York, NY

Jennifer A. Mathur, PhD
Clinical Director
Comprehensive Psychiatric Emergency
  Program (CPEP) Forensic
  Evaluation Service
Bellevue Hospital Center
Clinical Assistant Professor
Department of Psychiatry
New York University School
  of Medicine
New York, NY

Katherine Maloy, MD
Associate Director
Bellevue Comprehensive Psychiatric
  Emergency Program
Clinical Assistant Professor
New York University Department
  of Psychiatry
New York, NY

Didier Murilloparra, MD
Medical Student
New York University
  School of Medicine

Madeleine O'Brien, MD
Clinical Instructor
Department of Psychiatry
New York University School
  of Medicine
New York, NY

Dennis M. Popeo, MD
Unit Chief
Bellevue Geriatric Psychiatry
Associate Professor of Psychiatry
New York University School
  of Medicine
New York, NY

Amit Rajparia, MD
Director
Psychiatric Emergency Services
Bellevue Hospital Center
Clinical Associate Professor
  of Psychiatry
New York University School
  of Medicine
New York, NY

Yona Heettner Silverman, MD
Psychiatry Resident
New York University School
  of Medicine
New York, NY

Bipin Subedi, MD
Program Director
Forensic Psychiatry Fellowship
Clinical Assistant Professor
Department of Psychiatry
New York University School
  of Medicine
Attending Psychiatrist
Forensic Psychiatry Service
Bellevue Hospital Center
New York, NY

Jessica Woodman, MD
Psychiatry Resident
New York University School
  of Medicine
New York, NY

Daniel J. Zimmerman, MD
Psychiatrist in Private Practice
Clinical Instructor
Department of Psychiatry
New York University
New York, NY

Miriam Tanja Zincke, MD, MPH
Attending Psychiatrist
Bellevue Comprehensive Psychiatric
  Emergency Department
Clinical Instructor
New York University
  School of Medicine
New York University
New York, NY

Introduction

The term *emergency psychiatry* has a wide range of meanings and implications, and how emergency psychiatric care is provided may take many forms. Patients may present to the emergency department with an acute psychiatric complaint, they may arrive as walk-ins to an urgent care setting needing referrals and medication refills, they may present for a real or perceived medical issue and have unmet mental health needs driving their presentation, or they may be in the community with an acute, severe behavioral disturbance. Depending on the volume of patients, local mental health laws, availability of trained clinicians, and the design of the emergency department itself, emergency psychiatric care can be delivered in many ways. Some systems rely on an on-call clinician, possibly a psychiatrist, but at other times on a social worker or advanced practice nurse, who provides an evaluation and recommendations for treatment. Other systems with high volumes of patients in need of psychiatric care have developed more comprehensive emergency department–based services that include aftercare, short-term inpatient treatment, and extensive supportive services.

Still other systems, with more severe shortages of practitioners or where travel to the patient's location is a challenge, rely on telepsychiatry to provide consultation. In many health care systems there is a long wait for outpatient care, and it can be particularly difficult to access without insurance, outside of regular working hours, or due to transportation issues. Emergency medicine physicians will also note that many patients who present for issues related to chronic medical conditions also have ongoing mental health needs that are either contributing to their current visit or to their overall difficulties in maintaining their health outside the hospital.

Although comprehensive emergency psychiatric services or crisis centers are a way of meeting many of the challenges in providing immediate evaluation, diagnosis, and referral to appropriate treatment, they are certainly not the norm. Particularly in smaller, low-volume health care settings, there may not be sufficient volume to provide such depth of service. Emergency psychiatric care may fall on the shoulders of an emergency medicine physician or nurse practitioner. The clinician working at an urgent care center may be the first person to evaluate someone with new onset of serious mental illness or the first person to notice a substance use disorder. These clinicians may not feel they have sufficient training to intervene, or they may not be as eager to look for something they feel ill-equipped to manage. Similarly, although psychiatric residents are frequently called upon to cover emergency department consultation as part of their training, without sufficient support they may experience this work as overwhelming and unpleasant. Patients without adequate health care resources also disproportionately use emergency services over outpatient services, and thus the burden of comorbidity of medical problems, substance use disorders, and social issues such as homelessness or economic adversity may be high in the emergency setting.

Working in an emergency or urgent-care setting requires flexibility, a practical approach, and a broad range of knowledge. The ability to maintain calm in serious and confusing situations, to work in a team and as a consultant, to provide support and build an alliance not just with patients but with emergency department staff, and to make decisions with limited information are all important qualities. The work itself is rarely dull and provides the opportunity to keep up with one's "medical" training. Memorable cases can provide an anchor for clinical knowledge, whether for one's own education or for teaching. Toward that end, this book strives to draw on the authors' experiences as psychiatrists working in the emergency setting—but also their additional training in addiction, child, psychosomatic, and forensic psychiatry—to provide a case-based approach to problems that are frequently encountered in the emergency setting.

The cases in this book do not represent actual patients but are composites based on the experiences of the authors working in multiple settings. The situations described are designed to illustrate a range of issues, from more routine issues such as panic attacks and mild depression to more complex issues such as patients with severe personality disorders or neurologic issues that masquerade as behavioral problems. While many of the chapters deal specifically with groups of disorders—mood, anxiety, psychosis, personality, substance use, developmental disability—others delve into more complicated topics such as ethical obligations of the psychiatrist, working with patients in custody or who may commit crimes in the emergency department, or consulting to the medical emergency department about patients with somatization. The crossover between medical/neurologic illness and its behavioral manifestations is explored, as well as the impact of the clinician's own countertransference on evaluation and disposition. The case histories are punctuated by clinical tips and learning points that derive from the authors' experience, and they are followed by discussion that includes references to current literature and evidence-based practices. The topics covered should provide a broad knowledge base that clinicians working in emergency settings can refer to for clinical guidance in complicated situations and, we hope, spark an interest in this compelling and developing field.

Anxiety, Trauma, and Hoarding

KATHERINE MALOY ■

CASE 1: "I COULDN'T BREATHE"

Case History

Ms. D is a 26-year-old woman with no known prior psychiatric or medical history who presents to the psychiatric emergency department (ED) via ambulance after an episode of dyspnea on a train platform. The patient appears calm on arrival and does not understand why she has been triaged to the psychiatry side of the ED. She notes, "I couldn't breathe, what am I doing here in psych?" and states that she feels better anyway and needs to get to work.

The emergency medicine technician (EMT) accompanying the patient notes that when they arrived she was panting, flushed, and clutching her chest, stating she felt like she was going to die. Her lungs were clear, oxygen saturation was 100% on room air, and she denied any history of asthma, allergies, heart problems, or recent illness. A large crowd had gathered around the patient and so the EMTs rapidly moved her out of the train station and into the back of the ambulance where she could have some privacy. After a few minutes of controlled breathing directed by one of the EMTs, the patient's symptoms had resolved. She wanted to be transported to the hospital, however, because she was worried that something was medically wrong with her. When she arrived at triage with normal vital signs and no signs of distress, the nurse had decided that she had experienced a panic attack and sent her to the psychiatric side of the ED.

Clinical Tip

In a young patient with no signs of medical illness or comorbidity the likelihood that the patient is experiencing an acute MI or other medical illness is low, particularly since the symptoms resolved so quickly. However, once symptoms resolve, the patient may not wish to endure an evaluation in a psychiatric setting either, and may be reluctant to immediately identify his or her symptoms as psychiatric in nature.

Clinical Evaluation: The patient agreed to see the psychiatrist as long as she also is medically evaluated. On interview, the patient reports that she was on her way to work and thinking about her recent interactions with her supervisor when the symptoms began. She has been written up several times and is in danger of losing her job. She was already running late, and was anticipating getting "chewed out" by her boss once she got to work. She was running to catch the train and breathing rapidly. She has some financial problems already, and lives with her family as a result. She denied any depressed mood or other symptoms of depression but does note more difficulty concentrating at work and having over the past few weeks a few episodes where she begins thinking about all of her problems and "my mind just races and I feel like I'm going to pass out." She ate a good breakfast this morning, drank her usual one cup of coffee, and denies use of cigarettes, drugs, or alcohol. She saw her primary care doctor a few months ago and was deemed healthy but was advised to exercise more frequently. She denies having any history of suicide attempts, arrest, violence, or prior psychiatric hospitalizations.

On physical exam, no abnormalities are detected. Electrocardiogram is normal. Laboratory studies show no signs of metabolic problems, anemia, or thyroid disease. She submits urine for toxicology and no substances are detected. Urinalysis is normal. The psychiatrist reviews her chart and begins to think about how he is going to explain to Ms. D what happened to her.

"So, What's Wrong with Me? Is It All in My Head?"

While Ms. D is sitting in the psychiatric ED waiting for the results of her labs, a very agitated patient is brought by police in restraints. He is shouting, very malodorous, and accompanied by a crowd of police, EMS workers, and staff from the medical ED. Ms. D did not want to sit in the locked portion of the ED, so she is now sitting in the waiting area while the new patient is given sedating medications and restrained. The waiting area is suddenly very crowded. Ms. D begins to breathe rapidly and then gets up and is seen crying, stating "I've got to get out of here!"

Clinical Tip

Anxiety and panic can be precipitated by closed spaces, crowds, or stressful situations. Ms. D is likely having a panic attack precipitated by a situation not uncommon in a busy psychiatric ED.

Ms. D is moved to a quieter area, and one of the staff sits with her and helps her slow down her breathing. As soon as the acute crisis with the other patient is resolved, the psychiatrist meets with Ms. D to explain the likely diagnosis.

Ms. D is not totally convinced that there is not something medically wrong with her and reinforces several times to the psychiatrist that her heart was beating very quickly and that she "felt like my chest was thumping inside." Eventually she blurts out, "So I'm crazy? That's what it feels like, like I'm going crazy and I'm going to lose my mind and end up in the looney bin!"

The psychiatrist is able to reassure her that this does not mean she is in any way "crazy" and that the sensation of feeling "crazy" or out of control can in fact be a symptom of a panic attack. Ms. D is also able to recall some incidents from her late teens when she had similar symptoms. The patient was given referral information for treatment options, including cognitive behavioral therapy.

DISCUSSION

Panic attacks are a common precipitant for ED visits, particularly if patients do not understand what is happening to them, as the symptoms closely mimic an acute respiratory or cardiac problem. Rapid heart rate, rapid breathing, and the feeling of having "palpitations," being weak or faint, and of "impending doom" are all features that could be shared by many disorders. In a young and otherwise healthy patient with no comorbidities, the diagnosis of a panic attack can probably be mostly made by clinical history, most prominently by the fact that the classic symptoms should be self-limiting and resolve on their own.

Clinical Features and Epidemiology

Panic disorder is defined as recurrent, unexpected panic attacks that are either causing significant, distressing worry about having more attacks or leading to changes in behavior to avoid attacks for at least one month.[1] It is possible to have isolated panic attacks without meeting criteria for the disorder, as long as they are infrequent and not disabling. Median age of onset is 20 to 24 years, with new cases rarely diagnosed after 45 years of age.[2]

Differential diagnosis—apart from ruling out any acute medical causes of the symptoms—should also include an investigation into substance-related causes of anxiety symptoms and a thorough investigation into comorbid mood and psychotic symptoms. Patients may be more willing to report their symptoms as a "panic attack" than an adverse anxious or paranoid reaction to use of cannabis or stimulants. Withdrawal from alcohol or benzodiazepines can precipitate intense anxiety that may be identified by the patient as panic. Patients may also describe having "panic attacks" but their overall symptoms are more consistent with a generalized anxiety disorder. While it is difficult to make the diagnosis of a personality disorder in the ED, patients with borderline or histrionic traits may have episodes that they describe as panic or anxiety attacks when, in fact, they are more consistent with periods of emotional dysregulation.

The etiology of panic disorder is still not completely understood, but some researchers hypothesize a dysregulation of the normal fight or flight response to stressful stimuli and overactivation of a normal fear response.[3]

Panic Disorder and the Emergency Department

Although anxiety disorders in general are considered to be less serious than other mental disorders such as schizophrenia or bipolar disorder, panic disorder can be disabling, may lead to withdrawal from daily activities, and is associated with higher risk of suicide attempts in patients who also meet criteria for depression.[4] Undiagnosed or unrecognized panic disorder can also lead to excessive use of emergency medical services, as patients may appear as though they are having an acute medical issue or may believe, despite multiple workups, that they are having an undetected medical problem.[5] Worry begets worry, and the fear of having a panic attack may become even more disabling than the attacks themselves. Patients may withdraw from society to avoid triggers such as crowds, bridges, or elevators or be unable to complete basic daily activities due to their intense worry about having an attack or being embarrassed by their symptoms.

Most patients with panic disorder will not have a history of physical or sexual abuse, but patients who exhibit panic symptoms should be screened for posttraumatic stress disorder (PTSD), as there may be other symptoms of PTSD that are going unrecognized. An episode of reexperiencing a trauma or flashback could look like a panic attack in terms of autonomic hyperarousal and anxiety. Patients should also be screened for comorbid depression, as well as substance use disorders.

The good news is that panic disorder is quite treatable and can frequently be treated without medications.[6] For patients who are fearful that they are "crazy," the news that a short course of manualized cognitive behavioral therapy might ameliorate their symptoms is frequently reassuring. Some of these techniques can even be introduced in the ED and rehearsed with the patient, such as controlled breathing and progressive muscle relaxation. The news that panic attacks are self-limiting and not fatal can itself be helpful in helping patients address the fear of the attack.

Starting medications in the ED should ideally be avoided unless follow-up is immediately available. Although selective serotonin reuptake inhibitors are the first-line treatment for panic disorder,[7,8] they take time to be effective and any side effects in an already anxious patient can lead to early discontinuation or worsening of anxiety. A patient who has a less than ideal response to a medication prescribed in the ED may then be unmotivated to seek continued treatment or may doubt the accuracy of the diagnosis. While short-acting benzodiazepines are frequently used "as needed" for panic attacks, the onset of action of most agents, even alprazolam, is longer than the duration of most panic attacks. Short-acting benzodiazepines are also highly habit-forming and can cause rebound anxiety as they wear off. Comorbid substance use disorder greatly increases the risk of abuse of prescribed substances. There is also always a risk of patients who come to the ED endorsing panic symptoms specifically seeking benzodiazepines, as well as patients who are not in fact experiencing panic disorder but are experiencing anxiety in the context of withdrawal from abused substances such as alcohol, benzodiazepines, or barbiturates. Some patients may have also tried illicitly obtained benzodiazepines to ameliorate their symptoms, and they may be reluctant to reveal this information. For patients without comorbid substance use disorders who have intense fear of having another attack, simply having a small supply of a short-acting benzodiazepine available may have a positive effect in empowering them to not restrict their behavior in fear of having another attack. Patients should, however, be questioned about comorbid substance use disorders.

If a diagnosis of panic disorder can be made and conveyed to the patient effectively and the patient is able to engage in treatment, the result can be a great deal of savings in unneeded ED visits, health care costs, and a greatly improved quality of life for the patient.

Key Clinical Points

- Although medical comorbidities should always be considered, in young, otherwise healthy patients, panic disorder should be a consideration for patients with a classic cluster of symptoms.
- Other issues—apart from medical causes—that should be considered in the ED evaluation of panic attacks include adverse reaction to illicit drug use, seeking of prescriptions, and withdrawal from benzodiazepines or alcohol.
- Providing education about panic disorder and available treatment options can be helpful in reducing patient anxiety, avoiding overuse of medical services, and improving quality of life. Some brief interventions can be taught in an ER setting.

CASE 2: "STALLED IN THE HIGHWAY"

Case History

Initial Presentation: A 28-year-old white man is brought by ambulance and police from the middle of a highway. He was found standing next to a stalled delivery truck in the middle of traffic in a highly agitated state. Police had been called to help tow the truck out of traffic; on their arrival, the patient had become combative— arguing with police, demanding their rank, and wanting to speak to their commanding officer. Additional police and an ambulance were called to the scene. The man was restrained by several officers for transport to the hospital. One of the police noted that "It seemed like he was talking to people that weren't there . . . he kept calling me Sergeant." On arrival, the patient was diaphoretic, highly agitated, and tied to the stretcher. He did not seem to understand that he was speaking with a doctor. He appeared to be hallucinating. He was reciting military terminology. He was given intramuscular haloperidol and lorazepam, transferred to behavioral restraints, and he eventually fell asleep. Vital signs were notable for tachycardia on arrival but quickly returned to normal after sedation.

Routine laboratory studies were normal; alcohol level was zero. He was admitted to emergency observation. Pulse and blood pressure remained within normal limits consistently after sedation.

Learning Point: Evaluation of Altered Mental Status

The patient arrived in a highly agitated state, with abnormal vital signs and appearing disoriented to person, place, and time. While he appeared to be a young, healthy individual and vital signs rapidly normalized after sedation —suggesting that agitation was primarily responsible for his tachycardia—his presentation is concerning for a non-psychiatric etiology of his behavior. Monitoring of vital signs, laboratory studies, EKG, toxicology, and careful physical exam are all important initial interventions in this patient. A screening CT of the brain could be considered. Acute intoxication, particularly on a hallucinogenic compound or stimulant, would also be a leading diagnostic consideration.

Collateral Information: An hour after the patient arrived, a call was received from his employer, who had been notified by police. The patient had just begun a job as a delivery truck driver, and the employer noted he has a military background. The employer provided the patient's emergency contact number—that of his wife.

The patient's wife was contacted to attempt to obtain medical and psychiatric history. She reported no prior psychiatric history and was extremely concerned about his presentation. She noted that he had recently finished two years of military service in Iraq and that he had had difficulty finding a job. As a result the couple was under a great deal of financial stress. She denied that he uses drugs or alcohol, noting, "He's been looking for a job and every job requires a drug screen. He wouldn't mess that up."

Further Observation and Follow-Up: The patient woke overnight and was confused about his whereabouts but was calm and in control when informed of what had happened. He submitted urine for toxicology, which was negative for cocaine, barbiturates, opiates, phencyclidine, and THC but positive for benzodiazepines, which had been administered on arrival. He did not require any further sedation and his wife was notified at his request of his current condition. A CT scan of his head was obtained that did not reveal any space-occupying lesions, acute bleeds, or structural abnormalities.

Clinical Pearl: Reliability of Urine Drug Screens

Many patients conceal their use of drugs or alcohol for fear of judgment by providers, fear of prosecution, reporting to employers or child welfare officials, or simply due to stigma and shame. Despite reassurances from providers and sensitive, confidential interviewing, it may not be possible to obtain a fully honest substance use history. Some patients who are acutely intoxicated may be simply unable to provide any information. Toxicology screening for illicit substances can therefore be a useful tool when used in combination with clinical history. However, the types of screening available vary widely by hospital or laboratory, and turn-around times are not always rapid enough to be useful in the ER setting. Specimens are usually not obtained in an entirely secure manner; patients may be able to adulterate their urine with water or, in some extreme cases, switch it with that of another patient to avoid detection. Clinicians should also familiarize themselves with the expected window of time of a positive test for various substances and possible causes of false-positives (e.g., reports of dextromethorphan testing as phencyclidine), as well as false-negatives (e.g., some synthetic opioids not testing positive on a routine "opiates" screen).[9] Newer "designer" drugs are usually ahead of commercially available tests, as they are sometimes designed specifically to avoid commercially available testing (for example, synthetic cannabinoids or "bath salts").

The patient was re-interviewed in the morning by a psychiatrist and social worker. He was calm, polite, and deferential to staff, and he was extremely embarrassed about his behavior the day before. He insisted he was fine and denied all psychiatric symptoms; his thought process was linear and organized. He was quite fearful that he would lose his job as a result of this episode and wanted to leave as soon as possible to present to work and attempt to explain his behavior to his employer. There was no evidence of paranoia, thought disorder, or hallucinations. His wife came to the hospital to meet with the team and continued to deny witnessing any behavioral changes at home preceding the event. Both were reluctant to discuss any possible precipitants for the previous day's events, focusing instead on how important it was for the patient to stay employed.

On more extensive questioning, the patient discussed his military history. He spoke about driving a truck in Iraq and being constantly afraid of mines and ambushes. He spent most of his two years of service in situations where he was on constant alert. He had difficulty recalling the events of the day before, but he did recall being stuck on the bridge after his truck stalled, particularly the noise of the traffic, people in other cars yelling at him, and his feeling of intense panic that he was surrounded and could not get away. He had not been injured while in the military but had witnessed injuries to members of his company as well as hearing numerous stories of soldiers who were maimed or killed in situations similar to his. Since returning home, he admitted to having periodic nightmares, from which he wakes in a state of intense agitation. He reported difficulty remembering that he is no longer in Iraq, as well as times when he feels as though he is reexperiencing certain situations. He noted that he sometimes withdraws from his wife and does not speak to her about what he is experiencing, noting that he already feels guilty for their financial problems and does not want to burden her with his difficulties.

Learning Point: Differential Diagnosis

Upon ruling out a non-psychiatric medical etiology of the patient's presentation, as well as acute intoxication, more information must be gleaned about his recent history. There was no evidence of a prodromal period of worsening function, decline in self-care, or social withdrawal. There was no evidence either from the patient or his wife of an onset of hypomanic or manic symptoms. Although the patient admitted to feeling worried about his financial situation and sad at times when thinking about friends he had lost, he did not meet full criteria for a depressive episode or generalized anxiety disorder; there was no evidence of discreet panic attacks. Given that he had a very brief period of psychotic symptoms, brief psychotic disorder would be a consideration. However, brief psychotic disorder is characterized by a period of psychotic symptoms that lasts more than one day but less than one month, and it is characterized by at least two of the following: delusions, hallucinations, disorganized speech, or grossly disorganized behavior. The patient's symptoms lasted less than a few hours, and so he does not meet full criteria.

Once he was willing to discuss how his military service might be affecting him on a day-to-day basis, the patient more clearly met criteria for PTSD, with this episode representing a very dramatic and frightening flashback.[10] He described ongoing fear of loss of life for two years of service in war, as well as witnessing deaths of friends and close colleagues. He reported avoidance of situations that reminded him of his service, emotional numbing, distancing himself from family, and persistent negative cognitions about his difficulties and his service. He had experienced nightmares and hypervigilance with increased startle reflex. Stuck on a crowded bridge surrounded by noise, trucks, and angry drivers, he became overwhelmed. The patient's intense fear of losing his job and shame about his difficulties made it difficult to engage him in the evaluation and left him reluctant to seek treatment.

Disposition: The patient had no health insurance. He did not want to apply for veteran's benefits coverage, as he expressed fear that simply walking into a Veteran's Administration (VA) hospital to apply for benefits would cause intense anxiety and distress. He accepted a referral to follow-up onsite and was open to the idea that he may have experienced a flashback that was related to his prior military service and triggered by stress. He accepted a note clearing him to return to work, but he did not want anyone to contact his employer directly to discuss his symptoms.

DISCUSSION

Epidemiology and Clinical Features

PTSD is heterogeneous in its course and presentation and can masquerade as other psychiatric syndromes, as it can present with features of irritability, depressed mood, anhedonia, anxiety, panic, and even at times psychosis.[10,11] Onset can be delayed, and presence or absence of an acute stress reaction immediately after a trauma is not a reliable predictor of development of PTSD.[11,12] Risk factors include history of prior trauma, comorbid substance abuse, and preexisting psychiatric disorders.[13] Women have a higher rate of PTSD than men, one possible explanation being a higher rate of exposure to interpersonal violence and sexual assault.[14] In a study of a large community sample, PTSD was uniquely associated with disability, suicidality, and poor quality of life after correcting for other mental disorders.[15] Patients may not want to report symptoms due to stigma, fear of losing employment, avoidance of reliving the experience, fear of disclosure of comorbid drug or alcohol use, or simply due to the negative cognitions that can be part of the syndrome itself, that is, a belief that this is all the patient's own fault to begin with. In this case, the patient's fear of triggering traumatic memories coupled with his negative beliefs about his service in the military had led him to avoid a potential source of help, the VA Hospital.

Trauma-Related Disorders and the Emergency Department

The ED setting—as well as events leading up to arrival, such as police involvement, involuntary transportation by EMS, lights, sirens, loud vehicles, crowds—can all be factors in acutely worsening the condition of a patient with a history of trauma, regardless of whether they meet full criteria for PTSD. The setup of a psychiatric emergency setting can be specifically counter-therapeutic: EDs are frequently loud, other patients may be agitated, and staff who are attempting to maintain safety may be perceived as intrusive or aggressive. Patients with a history of trauma may not be able to verbalize their internal experience and may not effectively communicate their needs. For a woman with a history of physical or sexual trauma, for example, being in a confined space surrounded by male patients can be terrifying. Being placed in restraints or in a seclusion room is a last resort for patients who are acutely dangerous, but with someone with a history of physical or sexual trauma or forced confinement, it can precipitate symptoms such as flashbacks or intense panic. Patients who have been incarcerated before, and who have suffered trauma during their incarceration, are particularly triggered by locked doors and by many of the safety procedures that a psychiatric emergency service may consider routine, such as requirements for search, giving up clothes, going through metal detectors, metal detecting wands, body pat-downs, or in some settings, even strip searches. For the patient discussed in this case, the acute environment of police response to his stalled vehicle and arrival to the hospital surrounded by police, EMS, hospital workers and staff most likely worsened his acutely fearful state.

Evaluating psychiatric patients in the ED setting should include screening for a history of trauma—including sexual and physical abuse, interpersonal violence, and exposure to traumatic events—as well as military history. Although it may not be appropriate to delve into details of past abuses, it is nonetheless information that is an important part of diagnostic evaluation and a context in which to frame interventions for the patient. Interventions for managing the patient's behavior can then incorporate this information. For example, a woman with a history of sexual abuse might be provided with a more private space during evaluation away from male patients, or a patient who has an exaggerated startle response to loud noises might require a quieter setting or a voluntary stay in seclusion to de-escalate when feeling triggered. Evaluating for and responding to a patient's history of trauma is an important facet of providing patient-centered care.

Evidence-Based Treatment and Disposition

In terms of disposition and referral to aftercare, treatment of PTSD can be effective, but most patients still do not receive appropriate care.[16] Pharmacotherapy options include medication for depressive and anxiety-spectrum symptoms, as well as use of antipsychotic medication as augmentation if psychotic symptoms are persistent or prominent and specific anti-adrenergic agents to prevent the physiologic response to nightmares and improve sleep.[17] Psychotherapeutic interventions include cognitive-behavioral therapy, focusing on exposure and response prevention.[18] Prolonged exposure therapy has been shown to be efficacious, as well as reduce health care utilization in VA populations.[19] However, systematic reviews have been less conclusive in patients with chronic PTSD symptoms.[20,21] In this patient, who was reluctant to consider any medications, stressing psychotherapeutic, cognitive-based interventions may have been a way of engaging him in treatment. This patient had a supportive spouse and an employer who was aware of his military history and invested in hiring and retaining veterans—both positive prognostic factors in terms of being able to maintain financial independence and employment.[22]

Key Clinical Points

- Acute agitation can be caused by or worsened by a history of trauma, even if a patient does not meet full criteria for a trauma-related disorder.
- The ED setting itself can worsen or provoke symptoms in patients with history of physical, sexual, or emotional abuse and combat- or incarceration-related trauma. Providers should be vigilant about screening for history of trauma or abuse and attempt to provide accommodation for patients that minimizes triggers while still maintaining safety.
- Negative self-perceptions and cognitive distortion are part of the syndrome of PTSD, and may lead to difficulty reporting symptoms and minimizing triggers and shame, thus further limiting access to treatment.

CASE 3: "AN UNLIVABLE SITUATION"

Case History

Ms. B is a 66-year-old white woman who is brought by ambulance with police and adult protective services escort from her apartment a few blocks away from the hospital. She is angry and combative, wearing only a bathrobe and slippers despite cold temperatures outdoors and slapping at police who are attempting to bring her into the ED. Emergency medical services (EMS) workers escorting the patient state that the patient was "removed" today from her apartment by "social workers" and that the apartment is "unbelievably disgusting." They do not know her medical or psychiatric history because she has refused to cooperate with any assessment, including vital signs. They do not know what precipitated the removal today, as they were summoned by police on the scene after the patient refused to open her door. The lock was drilled to gain entry.

Once Ms. B arrived at the ED, she did cooperate with initial vital signs, which were not grossly abnormal: blood pressure of 142/80, pulse of 90, respirations of 16, and temperature 98.8. The patient even agreed to have a finger-stick glucose measurement which was 94. She denied having any chest pain or any other somatic symptoms but was angry and yelling, so psychiatry was called to evaluate her.

The patient cooperated with laboratory studies, which were all normal.

On interview, she does not have any idea why she is in the hospital and wants to return to her apartment immediately, as she notes that the people who "kidnapped" her today have moved some of her valuable antiques and may have caused damage to some of her important items. She refused to provide contact information for any friends or family. She is fully oriented to person, place, and time but refused any detailed cognitive screening.

Past Psychiatric History: The patient denies ever seeing a psychiatrist. There are no prior visits at the hospital where she is being seen.

Social History: She refuses to disclose much information apart from stating she supports herself selling antiques, and that she needs to return to her apartment immediately to make sure all of her items are intact. She denies use of tobacco, alcohol, or illicit drugs. She denies having any family or friends.

Medical History: She denies having any medical problems. She does not believe in "western medicine" and thus does not have a primary care doctor.

At this point, the patient has calmed down and is sitting quietly in her bathrobe and slippers, requesting to leave the ED. The consulting psychiatrist sets out to find out why the patient was brought to the ED in the first place.

Clinical Tip

The patient was removed from her home for reasons that remain unclear. Although she is now calm and reasonably organized, she does appear to have some indicators of poor self-care. In a situation where it is not clear why the patient was removed against her will to a hospital, even if the patient is currently appearing somewhat stable, further investigation is probably warranted.

The consulting psychiatrist transfers the patient to the psychiatric ED so as to prevent elopement while reasons for removal are investigated. In the patient's chart, there is a card for a social service agency. The psychiatrist manages to locate the caseworkers who accompanied the patient to the hospital, as well as a copy of the EMS and police reports that describe the condition of her apartment.

The caseworkers relate that they are working for adult protective services after a complaint was filed by the landlord of her building, alleging the patient is refusing to allow repair of a water leak, that awful odors were coming from the patient's apartment, and that no one in the building had actually seen her going outside in several months. Initially, the complaint was investigated and insufficient evidence was found to warrant breaking into her apartment. A second complaint was filed when the patient stopped paying her rent and was in eviction proceedings. The patient had also been seen stealing items out of the building garbage and bringing them into her apartment. A court order was obtained after multiple attempts to gain entry with the patient's consent.

Caseworkers describe an apartment currently without any running water or workable toilet. The patient has a small passageway where she can walk, with trash piled up to the ceiling in many places. She is urinating and defecating into a pot, which she periodically empties into the building trash chute. It was not clear to them on examining the apartment where she was sleeping. Mice were observed tunneling through the debris. When they opened the door and explained to the patient that she had to be evaluated and began moving some of the trash out of the way to allow the door to open fully, she became agitated and "hysterical" and EMS was summoned. They show pictures taken of the apartment that confirm all of their descriptions.

According to the caseworkers, if the patient allows them to work with her, they can prevent her from being evicted by providing money management, rent assistance, and cleaning services. She would have to allow them to help her apply for disability or show some other source of income to allow for rent payments ongoing, even if the court can provide a one-time grant for her rent arrears. She would also have to permit a deep-cleaning and fumigation, as neighbors are complaining of infestation in their apartments that cannot be ameliorated until her apartment is dealt with.

The psychiatrist returns to the patient to discuss all of this information with her. She insists that she is making plenty of money as an antique dealer and "things will pick up soon" once she is able to sell some more furniture. She asserts that all of the items in her apartment are "treasures" and that none of them can be thrown out. She will not permit anyone in her apartment, since they are likely to break important objects and ruin them for future use. She in fact becomes so agitated during this conversation that she cannot stop crying and shaking. She insists they are trying to steal her apartment and her valuable things.

To Admit or Not to Admit?

The decision of whether to admit this patient comes down to what a clinician's view is of her inability to safely care for herself. One could argue that by living in a filthy, vermin-ridden apartment where she has nowhere to even lie down, not leaving the house except to retrieve garbage, not bathing due to not having plumbing, she has reached the threshold of dangerously poor self-care. She is also in danger of losing her housing. In addition, one could argue that she is infesting her neighbors' apartments and putting them, as well as potentially the building's plumbing system and structural integrity, in danger. She is clearly delusional about the state of her apartment. However, one could also argue that the patient probably has lived like this for months to years, is not violent or suicidal, and has the right to choose the live the way she pleases. It may not in fact be unrealistic for her to believe that building management is trying to get her out of the building. In this case, it seemed that the landlord would have had an easier time evicting her if he had not involved social services, and he did in fact have her best interests at heart. Ideally, some compromise could be found to allow this patient to remain in the community while still keeping her safe.

Outcome: In this case, the patient was given 1 mg of oral lorazepam to help her calm down after she became agitated in the ED. She ended up requesting to stay overnight to "think things over" as she was also afraid to sleep in her apartment now that the lock was broken. She eventually agreed to allow the agency to enter her apartment as long as she was onsite when it occurred and to participate in a plan to avoid losing the apartment. She admitted that she would like to have a working toilet, although she blamed the landlord for breaking it on purpose. While she would not admit that there were any safety concerns, she was demonstrating a willingness to work on her situation in order to stay in the community, and adult protective services was able to arrange brief stay in a crisis respite unit. She was discharged to stay at the respite, with the plan that she would return back to her apartment with detailed social service plan to assist her in ameliorating the issues once basic safety issues were addressed.

DISCUSSION

Hoarding disorder is newly classified in DSM-V under "Obsessive Compulsive and Related Disorders." However, hoarding behavior can arise from many psychiatric conditions, and many hoarders are not obsessive or compulsive. Hoarding may not come to anyone's attention unless there is a consequence to neighbors, family, or friends. The Collyer brothers of New York City are famous for being crushed to death under their own hoarded garbage; ironically, their situation probably persisted long enough to allow death in this manner because they had sufficient resources to afford a building all to themselves.[23] In urban settings, where people live close together in apartment buildings, the consequences may be more immediately obvious: neighboring infestations, odors, visible trash glanced through an open door, or frank structural problems. However, in a more suburban or rural setting, hoarding may not reveal itself unless someone gets access to the residence, children are involved, a medical issue is discovered, or a separate issue arises, such as nonpayment of property taxes or exterior property disrepair.

Clinical Features and Differential Diagnosis

The differential diagnosis of hoarding behavior is broad. Although it is not likely to be used in an ED setting, as it is designed to be used in the patient's home or with accompanying photographic evidence, a structured diagnostic interview for hoarding disorder does exist, and it may help guide clinicians in approaching the subject with patients.[24] Hoarding can involve obsessive collection of objects; difficulty parting with objects, involving intense anxiety; and disruption of normal living conditions due to excessive collecting or inability to clean and organize. The hoarding may or may not cause conscious distress to the hoarder, and it may occur in someone who does not clearly meet criteria for any other psychiatric disorder. Hoarders may also meet criteria for other disorders such as depression, anxiety, attention deficit hyperactivity disorder (ADHD) or obsessive compulsive disorder (OCD).[25,26] Some hoarders clearly meet criteria for OCD. However, many other disorders can contribute to hoarding. Patients can hoard due to psychotic illness, either due to disorganization and negative symptoms or due to delusions about the hoarded material and its importance. Patients with dementia or cognitive impairments can hoard due to their inability to manage their environment, paranoia interfering with their willingness to allow assistance with daily living, or repetitive and rummaging behaviors seen in Alzheimer's patients. Someone with severe depression could allow their clutter to get out of control due to apathy and neurovegetative symptoms. A person with a complicated grieving process might be unable to let go of items related to the deceased loved one. Patients with autism spectrum disorders may hoard due to obsessive collections related to their narrow interests, and their impairment in social skills can contribute to difficulty recognizing the problem and its impact on others.[27] Patients with childhood trauma related to loss and abandonment may hoard food or other items to ward off fears of starvation or neglect.[28] It is not uncommon to see spouses who are accustomed to having the house managed by their partner, who is now cognitively or physically disabled, encased in clutter and debris as a result of the partner's disability and their own denial. Physically disabled persons who lack support can find themselves surrounded by clutter without any clear comorbid psychiatric illness simply due to their physical impairments. In some cases, chronic personality traits lead to social isolation, which promotes hoarding by eliminating normal social checks on excessive behaviors.

Hoarding and the Emergency Department

Because there is a lot of shame and isolation associated with hoarding behavior, patients with hoarding behavior usually do not end up in the ED seeking help of their own volition. Typical scenarios in which psychiatry may be consulted include the story related in this case, that is, when someone is removed from an unsafe situation, social services gets involved, or pending eviction. Patients may present only after eviction, when they have nowhere else to go, or the problem is only discovered when they call 911 for some other reasons, such as an acute medical issue.

Diagnosing the cause of the hoarding problem can assist in making a plan of action. If patients have a clear psychosis or mood episode contributing, treatment of the underlying disorder can help. However, most patients who have reached a point of hoarding and impaired living conditions sufficient to land them in a psychiatric ED will require additional support in the community to address the issue. Hospitalization alone is unlikely to solve the problem. While television shows about drastic interventions for hoarders have increased awareness of the issue, a one-time drastic clean-up is unlikely to cure hoarding behavior, and without maintenance and support, the clutter will creep back in. Patients may not require hospitalization but may be considered at risk of being unable to care for themselves in the community and require referral to adult protective services. If children are involved, referral to child protective services may be indicated as well. In most states, health care providers are mandated reporters of suspected child abuse or neglect; laws concerning reporting of adults are less clear, but clinicians working in an ED setting should familiarize themselves with local resources and the policies of their hospital or social work department on how reporting is handled.

Hoarders frequently do not accurately report the severity of their situation, either because of embarrassment or the disorder itself. Outside sources of collateral information are helpful in determining the true safety concerns and evaluating risk. A scale of hoarding severity has been developed that may assist in clarifying the severity of the problem.[29]

Prognosis

In this case the diagnosis remained somewhat unclear. The patient was delusional about her apartment's condition and the severity of her living conditions. She fancied herself an antiques dealer with rare items of great value, when in fact her apartment was filled with trash and rodents. She became anxious and terrified when her items were moved or touched. She denied having any close friends or family supports but was not receiving disability and had at some point supported herself, thus implying a work history. She did not clearly meet criteria for dementia, but refused some of the more nuanced cognitive testing. In summary, she seemed to have some anxiety and obsessional traits around her hoarding but also delusions, and she was possibly somewhat schizoid and paranoid in her personality, in that she was isolated and had no social supports. Without further history about her longitudinal functioning, it was not possible to arrive at a final diagnosis. One hopes that, over time, if she continued to work with social services agencies to make her apartment livable and to pay rent, more diagnostic information could be gathered. She remains, however, at high risk of losing her apartment. If the consultant had not pushed to investigate further, she might have returned to her apartment only to be evicted and end up homeless.

REFERENCES

1. Diagnostic and Statistical Manual of Psychiatric Disorders, 5th ed. "Anxiety Disorders." © American Psychiatric Association. http://dx.doi.org/10.1176/appi. books.9780890425596.dsm05

2. Kessler RC, Berglund P, Demler O, et al: Lifetime prevalence and age-of-onset distributions of DSM-IV disorders in the National Comorbidity Survey Replication. *Archives of General Psychiatry* 2005a; 62(6):593–602.

3. Gorman J, Kent J, Sullivan G, et al. Neuroanatomical hypothesis of panic disorder, revised. *American Journal of Psychiatry* 2014; 2(3):426–439. http://dx.doi.org/ 10.1176/foc.2.3.426

4. Katz D, Yaseen ZS, Mjtabai R, et al. Panic as an independent risk factor for suicide attempt in depressive illness, findings from the National Epidemiological Study on Alcohol and Related conditions. *Journal of Clinical Psychiatry* 2011; 72(12):1628–1635. doi:10.4088/JCP.10m06186blu

5. Klerman GL, Weissman MM, Ouellette R, et al. *Journal of the American Medical Association* 1991; 265(6):742–746. doi:10.1001/jama.1991.03460060074027

6. Otto MW, Deveny C. Cognitive behavioral therapy and treatment of panic disorder: Efficacy and strategies. *The Journal of Clinical Psychiatry* 2005; 66:Suppl 4:28–32.

7. Working Group on Panic Disorder. Practice guideline for the treatment of patients with panic disorder. *American Journal of Psychiatry* 1998; 155:Suppl1–348.

8. Otto MW, Tuby KS, Gould RA, McLean RY, Pollack MH. An effect-size analysis of the relative efficacy and tolerability of serotonin selective reuptake inhibitors for panic disorder. *American Journal of Psychiatry* 2001; 158:1989–1992.

9. Rainey PM. Laboratory principles. In Nelson LS, Lewin NA, Howland M, Hoffman RS, Goldfrank LR, Flomenbaum NE. eds. *Goldfrank's toxicologic emergencies*, 9e. New York, NY: McGraw-Hill; 2011. http://accessemergencymedicine.mhmedical.com.ezproxy.med.nyu.edu/content.aspx?bookid=454&Sectionid=40199370. Accessed September 3, 2014.

10. Trauma and stress related disorders. In: *Diagnostic and Statistical Manual of Psychiatric Disorders*, 5th ed. doi: 10.1176/appi.books.9780890425596.991543

11. Dickstein BD, Suvak M, Litz BT, et al. Heterogeneity in the course of posttraumatic stress disorder: Trajectories of symptomatology. *Journal of Trauma and Stress* 2010; 23(3):331–339.

12. Bryant, RA. Acute Stress Disorder as a predictor of posttraumatic stress disorder: A systematic review. *Journal of Clinical Psychiatry* Feb 2011; 72(2):233–239. doi: 10.4088/JCP.09r05072blu. Epub Dec 14 2010.

13. Bryant RA, Creamer M, O'Donell ML, Silove D, McFarlane AC. A multisite study of the capacity of acute stress disorder diagnosis to predict posttraumatic stress disorder. *Journal of Clinical Psychiatry* Jun 2008; 69(6):923–929.

14. Breslau N. The epidemiology of trauma, PTSD, and other posttrauma disorders. *Trauma Violence Abuse* Jul 2009; 10(3):198–210 doi: 10.1177/1524838009334448. Epub Apr 30, 2009.

15. Sareen J, Cox BJ, Stein MB, Afifi TO, Fleed C, Asmundson GJ. Physical and mental comorbidity, disability and suicidal behavior associated with posttraumatic stress disorder in a large community sample. *Psychosomatic Medicine* 2007; Apr(3):242–248. Epub Mar 30, 2007.

16. Kessler RC, Chiu WT, Demler O, Walters EE. Prevalence, severity, and comorbidity of twelve-month DSM-IV disorders in the National Comorbidity Survey Replication (NCS-R). *Archives of General Psychiatry* Jun 2005; 62(6):617–627.

17. Posttramatic stress disorder and acute stress disorder. In: Sadock B, Sadock V, Ruiz P eds., *Kaplan and Sadock comprehensive textbook of psychiatry.* Philadelphia: Lippincott, Williams and Wilkins, 2012: 258–263.

18. Ursano R, Bell C, Spencer E, et al. *Practice guidelines for treatment of patients with acute stress disorder and posttraumatic stress disorder.* Arlington, PA: American Psychiatric Association, 2004. DOI: 10.1176/appi.books.9780890423363.52257

19. Tuerk PW, Wangelin B, Rauch SA, et al. Health service utilization before and after evidence-based treatment for PTSD. *Psychology Series* 2013; 10(4):401–409. doi: 10.1037/a0030549. Epub Nov 1, 2012.

20. Hetrick SE, Purcell R, Garner B, Parslow R. Combined pharmacotherapy and psychological therapies for post traumatic stress disorder (PTSD). *Cochrane Database Systematic Review* Jul 7, 2010;7; 7:CD007316. doi: 10.1002/14651858.CD007316.pub2.

21. Bisson JL, Roberts NP, Andrew M, Cooper R, Lewis C. Psychological therapies for chronic post-traumatic stress disorder (PTSD) in adults. *Cochrane Database Systematic Review* Dec 13, 2013; 12:CD003388. doi: 10.1002/14651858.CD003388.pub4.

22. Karstoft KL, Armour C, Elklit A, Solomon Z. Long-term trajectories of posttraumatic stress disorder in veterans: The role of social resources. Journal of Clinical Psychiatry Dec 2013;74(12):e1163-8. doi: 10.4088/JCP.13m08428

23. Weiss K. Hoarding, hermitage and the law: Why we love the Collyer brothers. *Journal of American Academy of Psychiatry and the Law* 38(2): 251–257.

24. Norsletten AE, Fernandez de la Cruz L, Pertusa A, et al. The structured interview for hoarding disorder (SIHD): Development, usage and further validation. *Journal of Obsessive Compulsive and Related Disorders* 2013; 2(3): 346–350.

25. Obsessive-compulsive and related disorders: Hoarding. *Diagnostic and statistical manual of mental disorders,* 5th ed. Accessed electronically May 1, 2015. http://dx.doi.org/10.1176/appi.books.9780890425596.dsm06

26. Frost R, Steketee G, Tolin D. Comorbidity in hoarding disorder. *Depression and Anxiety* 2011; 28:876–884.

27. Pertusa A, Fonseca A. Hoarding in other disorders. *Oxford Handbook of Hoarding and Acquiring.* New York: Oxford University Press, 2014: 59–74.

28. Przeworski A, Cain N, Dunbeck K. Traumatic life events in individuals with hoarding symptoms, obsessive compulsive symptoms and comorbid obsessive and hoarding symptoms. *Journal of Obsessive-Compulsive and Related Disorders* 2014; 3:52–59.

29. Saxena S, Ayers C, Dozier M, Maidment M. The UCLA Hoarding Severity scale: Development and validation. *Journal of Affective Disorders* April 2015; 175:488–493.

2

Mood Disorders

Clinical Examples and Risk Assessment

JENNIFER GOLDMAN ■

CASE 1: "TOO WORRIED TO WAIT"

Case History

History of Present Illness: Mr. D is a 29-year-old man, employed and domiciled with his wife and daughter, with history of self-reported "anxiety and depression," who brings himself into the ED reporting worsening "stress" over past few weeks. On interview, the patient is dysphoric and tearful and reports noticed low mood, poor concentration, increased anxiety, and difficulty falling asleep over the past few weeks. Mr. D states that he recently restarted his "old supply" of Zoloft 50 mg, which he was breaking in half to "stretch it out until I found a doctor." He scheduled a new patient appointment with a primary care doctor for next week, but "got real low" the past few days and he "was too worried" to wait until his appointment. He describes feeling shame about his depression and his ambivalence about meeting with a "mental health doctor ... because I'm not crazy." He states that his wife is very supportive of him and of his getting treatment.

He reports some chronic passive thoughts of "not wanting to be alive" but denies any intent or plan to harm himself. He denies any history of acting on these thoughts. He states that his wife and daughter, as well as his religious faith, keep him from ever hurting himself. He denies violent ideation, hallucinations, or paranoid ideation. He reports smoking marijuana approximately once per week, and denies other substance use.

Mr. D was assessed using the Columbia Suicide Severity Rating Scale clinical practice screener (CSSRS).[1] He answered yes to one out of six questions (that he had had some wish for death over the past month) but answered no to having any suicidal thoughts, specific thoughts with a method, whether he had taken any steps toward harming himself, had any intent of harming himself, or had a history of suicidal behavior.

Collateral was obtained from patient's wife, who denies having any safety concerns about the patient. She reports a history of the patient's symptoms that is consistent with what patient reported. She says that the patient "knows himself and knows when to ask for help." She was aware that he was coming to the ER today and plans to meet him here shortly.

Past Psychiatric History: The patient reports he was prescribed antidepressant medication by his primary care doctor in Texas in the past. He took 100 mg sertraline daily for approximately one year and then discontinued it two years ago. The sertraline alleviated his depressive symptoms, and he had no side effects. He has no other past psychiatric treatment. He denies having any history of self-harm, suicide attempts, violence, or psychiatric hospitalization.

Substance Use History: He reports heavy marijuana use in his early 20s but states that since his daughter was born he uses it once a week at most.

Medical History: He denies history of medical problems. No major past hospitalizations.

Social/Developmental: The patient completed high school and works as a personal trainer at a gym. He lives with his wife and 3-year-old daughter. The family moved to New York City 3 months ago from Texas to be closer to his wife's family, who are helping with child care while the patient and his wife are working.

Family History: The patient had no family history of suicide. He has a paternal uncle with alcohol dependence.

Laboratory Studies: The patient completed blood work and EKG; there were no abnormalities found. Urine toxicology was positive for marijuana.

To Admit or Not to Admit?

Mr. D has depressed mood and occasional marijuana use. He has some passive suicidal thoughts, but no active ideation, plan, or intent; no history of self-harm; and has taken no preparatory steps toward suicide. He has strong family support and available follow-up in a few days with his primary care doctor. He has no medical problems that will interfere with his outpatient treatment and has a history of a good response to pharmacotherapy with no complications. The patient does not want to be admitted, and he does not require admission at this time based on all available information.

Disposition: Mr. D was not admitted to the hospital. Psychoeducation was provided to Mr. D and his wife about his diagnosis and his treatment options, including both psychotherapy and medication options. The patient's concern about the stigma related to mental health diagnoses and treatment was addressed and explored. His preference was to start outpatient treatment rather than inpatient treatment, as he was focused on wanting to return home to his wife and daughter and not wanting to miss any work. His wife was in agreement with his preference to start outpatient therapy and medication management. He was set up with an appointment for treatment in the mental health clinic for the following week. Given that his lab work and EKG were normal, that he had history of good response to sertraline, and that he was planning to continue his care at the evaluating hospital's clinic, he was given a 2-week prescription for sertraline 50 mg daily. Mr. D and his wife were encouraged to return to the ED if the patient's symptoms worsened, and they were also given other resources for mental health treatment in the community. Mr. D attended his first appointment and was enrolled in the hospital's outpatient mental health clinic.

CASE 2: "WHAT'S THE POINT?"

Case History

History of Present Illness: Ms. S is a 58-year-old woman, with a history of major depressive disorder, who is brought into the ED by her neighbor for evaluation. The neighbor shares concerns about the patient's increasingly isolative behavior and poor self-care over the past month. The neighbor states that although she doesn't know the patient very well, she knows that the patient lives alone. The neighbor became concerned earlier today when she heard the patient crying loudly and heard glass breaking. She knocked on the patient's door and convinced her to come to the ED.

On interview, Ms. S is initially only minimally cooperative, appearing guarded. She has a constricted, dysphoric affect and shows poor grooming. The patient admits that despite taking her Celexa 40 mg daily and Trazodone 100 mg at bedtime, she has noticed worsening of her depression over the past few months and recently feels "what's the point, it keeps coming back no matter what I do." She references prior depressive episodes in the past and states "this time it is the worst." She describes a worsening ability to sleep, lack of appetite, and a 10–15 lb. weight gain over past month. She reports multiple stressors, including losing her job 9 months ago, subsequently losing her health insurance, and facing possible eviction from her apartment. Furthermore, she is experiencing worsening pain from her arthritis.

Ms. S initially denies having any suicidal thoughts, but later admits to searching on the internet for painless ways to kill herself last night. She also researched which of her prescription pills could kill her if she overdosed and started to gather her pill bottles today prior to her neighbor visiting. She starts crying in the interview, stating that she had planned to overdose on all of her pills today.

Ms. S was assessed using the CSSRS. Her score is 5/6. She both wishes she would die and has active suicidal thoughts. She worked out a plan in detail, and has taken steps to accumulate a lethal amount of pills, as well as research exact doses. She had the intent of acting on those plans if she had not been interrupted by her neighbor's calling for help. She does not have a history of self-harm.

She denies homicidal ideation, hallucinations, or manic symptoms. There is no evidence of delusional thoughts on exam.

Collateral information is obtained from the patient's outpatient psychiatrist, who states that Ms. S is seen about once a month, but she missed her last appointment. He has been working with her for about a year and has noticed a recent worsening of her depressive symptoms over the past 3 months. He recently increased her citalopram to try and address the worsening symptoms.

Past Psychiatric History: The patient reports outpatient treatment for depression in the past. She describes three or four prior depressive episodes, which had been responsive to antidepressant medication and outpatient therapy. She most recently restarted treatment, two years ago, after the death of her husband. She has no history of psychiatric hospitalizations, no history of self-harm or suicide attempts, and no history of violence.

Substance Use History: Ms. S denies history of substance abuse. She reports drinking wine 2–3 times per month, usually one glass.

Medical History: She has a history of rheumatoid arthritis, currently stable, and is not currently on any steroids or other medications. She has no past hospitalizations.

Social/Developmental: Ms. S completed college and worked as a bank teller until nine months ago when she was laid off. She was married for 20 years until her husband passed away two years ago from cancer. She has no children. She identifies her church community as a source of friendships and support. She has no health insurance as a result of losing her job.

Family History: Ms. S's father committed suicide when she was in college. She is not sure of his psychiatric diagnosis.

Laboratory Studies: The patient agrees to blood work including CBC, BMP, LFTs, TSH, B12, and folate and RPR. All were normal. Urine toxicology was negative for substances.

Clinical Pearl: Voluntary versus Involuntary Admission?

In an emergency psychiatric evaluation, the psychiatrist will need to decide whether inpatient or outpatient treatment is appropriate. Some hospitals may have a broader variety of options than others—for example, admission to an extended observation unit or to a partial hospital program, in addition to an inpatient unit or an outpatient provider. The treatment setting decision will be based on the patient's examination, clinical formulation, and risk assessment. If an inpatient level of treatment is indicated, the decision to hospitalize a patient voluntarily versus involuntarily will depend on multiple factors, including the estimated level of risk to the patient and others, the patient's level of insight and willingness to seek care, and the legal criteria in that state. Given this, it is important for psychiatrists to be familiar with their specific state statutes regarding involuntary hospitalization.[2] As with other aspects of the evaluation, it is important to document the rationales for the decision you make regarding involuntary or voluntary psychiatric admission.

Disposition: Ms. S was admitted to the hospital on a voluntary status. Although she would have met criteria for involuntary commitment given imminent risk of harm to self,[3] the least restrictive means was pursued. She was assessed as having capacity to understand that she was admitting herself to a locked unit for treatment of a depression.

During her interview, she admitted that a barrier to her reaching out for help earlier (whether to her psychiatrist or by going to a hospital) was her concern about her loss of health insurance and worsening financial constraints. Her loss of insurance was part of why she did not attend her last appointment with her psychiatrist; she feared she would not be able to pay. She was relieved to hear that treatment at the hospital was available to her even without current health insurance, and she was assisted with an emergency Medicaid application to cover the hospital stay. When signing voluntary paperwork, she wrote, "I need help with depression so I do not commit suicide," as her reason for admitting herself to the hospital.

CASE 3: "I'M GREAT!"

Case History

History of Present Illness: Mr. F is a 36-year-old man, domiciled with a girlfriend and employed as a lawyer, with history of depression who was brought in by his girlfriend for concerns that he hasn't slept for 3 days. He reports that after experiencing depression for a few months he recently saw a psychiatrist and started taking an antidepressant medication. He says that for the past 2 weeks he has been feeling "remarkably better." His girlfriend shared concern that in addition to not sleeping, he "seems to have too much energy, he can't calm down and is talking a mile a minute!" On interview, patient displays pressured speech but is generally able to remain in good behavioral control. He is cooperative with assessment, describes his mood as "great," denies suicidal or violent ideation, and shows no evidence of delusional thought. He appears easily distracted and loses his train of thought frequently. He has some psychomotor agitation, tapping his foot throughout the interview. He denies suicidal or violent ideation, although he admits that he has been more irritable at work and he "almost got into a fist-fight there yesterday."

The patient scored 0/6 on the CSSRS.

Mr. F reports that his next appointment with his psychiatrist is next week and that he didn't call his doctor because he didn't feel there was any reason for concern. His psychiatrist was contacted for collateral. The psychiatrist had no knowledge of any of the patient's new symptoms and recommended that as long as there were no significant safety concerns, the patient should stop the medication and see him for a follow-up appointment the following day.

Past Psychiatric History: The patient reports one prior psychiatric hospitalization at age 18 for depression and grief after his mother passed away. He cannot recall what medication he took at that time but states he stopped it after about 2 months and has not been in any psychiatric treatment until recently. He has no history of self-harm, suicide attempts, or violence. He denies any past manic or psychotic episodes.

Substance Use History: He reports drinking alcohol 1–2 times per week "socially" and usually drinks one or two glasses of wine.

Medical History: He reports having mild hypertension but has not been prescribed antihypertensive medication. He also reports having both his tonsils and appendix removed while a teenager.

Social/Developmental History: The patient works at a large law firm, lives with his girlfriend, and has one child from a previous marriage with whom he visits regularly.

Family History: He reports his father has history of depression and his cousin has bipolar disorder.

Laboratory Studies: The patient's lab reports were unremarkable; urine toxicology was negative, as was ETOH level.

To Admit or Not to Admit?

Mr. F has not yet displayed any overtly dangerous behavior and he is not suicidal; however, he seems to have features of an emerging hypomania, and there is potential that his behavior will worsen. He would currently not meet criteria for an involuntary admission in most states. His symptoms could probably be managed in an outpatient setting if he has close follow-up.

Disposition: Mr. F showed limited insight into his current symptoms but was responsive to his girlfriend's concerns. With his permission, Mr. F's girlfriend was included in the discussion of his assessment and treatment options. Psychoeducation was provided to patient and his girlfriend about the likelihood that the patient was experiencing a hypomanic episode, possibly triggered by his antidepressant medication. He was offered inpatient admission but he declined. His preference was to stop the medication and follow up with his outpatient psychiatrist. As he did not endorse any suicidal or violent ideation, showed appropriate behavioral control, had not engaged in any dangerous or self-injurious behaviors, and showed adequate reality testing and motivation to continue psychiatric treatment, he did not meet criteria for involuntary commitment. The fact that this patient also had close outpatient follow-up to which he could return also helped mitigate the risk of an emerging hypomania.

Warning signs to return to the ED were reviewed with the patient and his girlfriend, and information was provided to them about support groups for patients and loved ones of those with mental illness. After further discussion, the patient's girlfriend was agreeable with the plan for discharge, and an appointment was set up with his psychiatrist. The girlfriend asked for recommendations for support; she was provided information on national and local resources for loved ones of those with mental illness. The patient was discharged with an appointment to see his psychiatrist the following day.

CASE 4: "I OWN THAT HOTEL!"

Case History

HISTORY OF PRESENT ILLNESS

Ms. Z is a 23-year-old woman with a history of bipolar disorder who was brought in by EMS from a hotel, after hotel staff called police reporting erratic behavior in the lobby. On triage, the patient was noted to be disheveled, loud, pacing the area, and yelling about being brought in to the ED, "I own that hotel, how dare you!"

On interview, she exhibits pressured speech, grandiose delusions (reports owning multiple hotels, as well as owning a television station) and psychomotor agitation. She is intense and irritable, and her behavior varies between crying and laughing throughout the exam. She denied any psychiatric complaints, stating: "I'm the best I've ever been!" She denied taking any psychiatric medication and denied any recent substance use. After the interview, she was observed being intrusive with other patients in the ER, and when staff approached her, she became assaultive. She required IM medication for safety.

Ms. Z had provided her parents' phone number as an emergency contact on arrival; she was informed that they would be contacted for collateral information. Her parents report that the patient has been missing for a week, after she left home saying she was accepted onto a reality television show. They were very worried about the patient's leaving but were unable to stop her. They state that she has spent all of her savings (approximately $8,000) within the past week.

The patient scored 0/6 on the CSSRS. She was quite irritable about the questions, stating "Why would I want to die? I'm amazing."

Past Psychiatric History: Ms. Z denies past psychiatric treatment, despite hospital records showing two prior inpatient psychiatric admissions for manic episodes. Her parents report that she was diagnosed with bipolar disorder at age 19. She was supposed to be attending outpatient therapy and was last taking lithium but has been noncompliant. She has no history of self-harm or suicide attempts. She has history of assaulting a family member during one of her prior manic episodes.

Substance Use History: Though she denies substance use on interview, she has remote history of cocaine and alcohol use. Per family, as far as they know, the patient last used substances over 2 years ago. Her urine toxicology on prior visits has been negative.

Medical History: No medical problems.

Social/Developmental: The patient left college after her first year and has been living with her parents since. She has had difficulty holding down a job and has been mainly supported by her family.

Family History: Her maternal grandmother and aunt both had been given diagnoses of bipolar disorder.

Laboratory Studies: Results include mildly elevated BUN and creatinine, likely to be secondary to dehydration. Urine toxicology is negative and blood alcohol level is zero.

To Admit or Not to Admit?

Ms. Z has demonstrated behavior that is clearly dangerous to others (assaulting staff in the ED) and indicates that she is unable to care for herself (agitated behavior in the community requiring police involvement, excessive spending). She also seems to lack any insight into her behavior.

Disposition: Ms. Z was admitted involuntarily to the inpatient psychiatric unit. She was felt to be an imminent danger to self and others as evidenced by her erratic and dangerous behavior, delusional thoughts influencing her behavior, poor insight, and judgment, behavior that would probably meet involuntary hospitalization requirements in most states.[2] She has a history of bipolar disorder and, likely due to her recent medication noncompliance, is presenting in an acutely manic and psychotic state. She spent two weeks on the inpatient unit being treated with mood stabilizing and anti-psychotic medication, after requiring a court order to provide medication over her objection.

DISCUSSION

The evaluation of patients with acute and chronic mood disorder symptoms is a common and critical part of any psychiatric emergency service. Because of the wide range of the variety and severity of symptoms, as well as the differing circumstances in which patients present, there is much to be considered when evaluating patients who present with depressive, manic, or hypomanic symptoms.

Safety

Given the nature of an emergency room, patients will frequently present in crises, and safety is a top priority. Patients with a history of mood disorder may present with acute manic or depressive symptoms. If manic, patients may exhibit agitated, dangerous behavior toward others. If acutely depressed or manic, patients may be brought in following self-injury or a suicide attempt. Prior to your assessment, it is crucial to establish safety for the patient and for others. This process should include a search of the patient (to ensure there are no objects that could cause harm) and may include giving emergent medication or placing the patient on close or 1:1 observation.[4] Finding a safe environment for patients to be evaluated in the medical ED setting that does not have separated psychiatric facilities can be particularly challenging.

For patients that present with severe agitation or disorganized behavior, an assessment should be held in an environment where clinicians can remove themselves if needed. As seen in the fourth case, patients may require emergent medication when verbal redirection is unsuccessful in protecting the patient or others from harm.[4] It is also important to obtain vital signs (including a finger-stick glucose), blood work (including a blood alcohol level), and toxicology, as these results will aid in determining an acute medical or substance-induced etiology.[5]

For patients that present following self-injury or reports of suicidal behavior, it is important to ensure that they, too, are medically stable. This may include checking for any recent ingestions or overdoses or assessing any wounds or trauma to make sure they do not require further medical intervention. Patients with severe depression, as in the second case, may also present in the context of poor self-care, possibly with poor intake of food or liquids. For these reasons, vital signs and blood work are essential components of your initial psychiatric evaluation.[5]

Differential Diagnosis

The presentation of patients with symptoms of a mood disorder is a frequent occurrence in a psychiatric emergency room setting. It is important to keep your differential wide, as you assess the type and severity of symptoms, gather information about the patient's history, and order necessary tests (blood work, urine toxicology, etc.) before completing your evaluation. Patients presenting for emergency psychiatric evaluation are known to have a high prevalence of combined general medical and psychiatric illness, recent trauma, substance-related conditions, and/or cognitive impairment. Frequently, a patient may present with symptoms of mania or depression that are secondary to causes other than major depressive disorder or bipolar disorder. Medical and substance-induced symptoms should always be considered. Patients with history of personality disorders may present with depressive or manic-like symptoms in the context of an acute stressor. A comprehensive evaluation is crucial, even for those with a known history of prior presentations for or treatment of a mood disorder.[2]

In an acute setting like the ED, timely assessments are crucial. Direct observation of the patient, information gathered from the interview with the patient, and the mental status examination will aid in diagnosis, as will collateral information from a patient's physicians, therapists, case workers, family, or friends. When available, past medical and psychiatric treatment history can aid in assessment and diagnosis. Important sources of information, apart from information obtained from the patient, include family or other collateral contacts, the medical record, or a referral letter or EMS report.[6]

The length of an emergency evaluation can vary greatly and often can exceed several hours. At some hospitals, a short-term observation unit is available in the emergency department for longitudinal observation, crisis stabilization, or substance metabolism. The evaluation may also vary depending on the time of day. Evening or overnight evaluations may be restricted by a limited ability to get collateral information from treatment providers or by the limited ability to set up outpatient follow-up.[5]

Emergency Psychiatry's Ever-Expanding Role

The psychiatric emergency room's role has grown increasingly varied and broad over the years. At its core, it remains a source of assessment and acute intervention when a patient's symptoms become intolerable to them or when their behaviors become worrisome to others. In the case of patients with mood disorders, this regularly includes severe depression, manic, or hypomanic symptoms. As outlined in their *Practice Guideline for the Psychiatric Evaluation of Adults*, the American Psychiatric Association highlights many of the important aspects of an emergency evaluation. These include establishing safety for the patient and others and identifying a provisional cause responsible for the current crises, including any possible medical or substance-related etiologies. When possible, the emergency room treatment team will identify and collaborate with any family, friends, or treatment providers who can aid in clarifying a history of events or symptoms, as well as aiding in treatment planning. This is particularly important for patients who are brought in against their will or those who are too agitated or cognitively impaired to provide information. After you have assessed for and established safety and organized your differential and risk assessment, the treatment team will need to work with the patient (and others) to develop a specific plan for disposition including either inpatient or outpatient follow-up.[6]

Due to a number of factors, the psychiatric ED's role has grown far beyond just emergent assessments. It has increasingly become a main entry point for people as they attempt to establish psychiatric care or as a resource for addressing psychosocial stressors that may be exacerbating their psychiatric condition.[7] It is not uncommon for patients to present to psychiatric EDs asking for help with access to care, referrals for mental health or substance abuse treatment, or medication prescriptions.

Examples of non-emergent reasons for patients with depression or bipolar disorder to present to the ED include a loss of previous treatment provider, a lapse in insurance coverage, or relocation to a new city or town. As illustrated in the first case, patients frequently receive treatment for mood disorders in the primary care setting. Patients may be referred to the ED from primary care offices when patients present there with more acute or severe psychiatric symptoms that are beyond the comfort or training of the primary care physician.

Both structural and attitudinal barriers to mental health treatment may deter patients from entering into treatment prior to their symptoms reaching the level of a crisis, thus leading to their emergency room presentation. It is important to understand these barriers when making your evaluation, as well as when planning for treatment and disposition.

Structural barriers include cost of treatment, lack or insufficient insurance coverage of mental health treatment, and difficulty getting outpatient appointments or being seen quickly enough.[7]

As a result, it is not uncommon for patients to present to EDs asking to be restarted on psychiatric medication or to obtain medication refills after having difficulty starting or restarting outpatient treatment through other means. Patients that were previously stable in outpatient treatment may present with an acute worsening of symptoms after treatment noncompliance or a loss of access to treatment. As illustrated in the second case, the patient's perceived lack of treatment options due to a loss of insurance/financial constraints probably contributed to the worsening of her depression and subsequent hospitalization.

Attitudinal barriers exist as well, including beliefs that mental health treatments are ineffective and an overall stigma about psychiatric diagnosis or treatment.[8] The psychiatric emergency room is a unique and important setting to provide psychoeducation to both patients and their families about diagnosis, prognosis, and available treatment options. The first case illustrates an example of someone who, due to shame about their symptoms and diagnosis, was hesitant to seek mental health treatment—"because I'm not crazy." Such people may go untreated or undertreated for years until their symptoms reach a point of crises. The ED setting may be their first interaction with trained mental health professionals. Because the mental health professional built a therapeutic alliance with this patient, the patient was willing to try outpatient therapy and see a psychiatrist for treatment of his depression.

As evident in the third case, involving a patient's family in his or her assessment and disposition plan aids in both treatment and safety planning. This allows for the opportunity to provide psychoeducation and resources not only to the patient but also directly to the family. Although the patient in the third case was already in psychiatric treatment prior to his emergency room presentation, he presented with new symptoms that affected his diagnosis and treatment options. Psychoeducation for this patient (and, with his permission, his girlfriend) about his diagnosis, prognosis, and treatment options was a critical part of the emergency room intervention, particularly given his preference to continue treatment in the outpatient, rather than inpatient, setting. Helping patients and their families understand the warning signs for when to take as-needed medication, when to call their doctor, or when to return to the ED are all important parts of a safe discharge plan.

A patient's experience in the psychiatric emergency room can affect the probability of their continuing treatment or the likelihood of their seeking emergency help in future times of crises. Crisis intervention is often necessary in the emergency room setting; however, as described by Ronald Rosenberg MD in his article titled "Psychological Treatments in the Psychiatric Emergency Service," family therapy, brief psychotherapy, and even cognitive therapy can be helpful interventions.

Addressing a patient's concerns about stigma, treatment ambivalence, and utilizing motivational interviewing can all improve patient outcomes.[9] Of note, these types of interventions can only be integrated when a patient is stable enough to participate. It is important to look at factors such as insight, reality testing, and mood stability when assessing the appropriateness of patients.

For patients presenting with mood disorders, psychiatric mediations should be used in the emergency room for three main purposes—to ensure patients are able to remain safe, to address acute distressing symptoms, and to initiate longer-term treatment. When patients present to the ED and are acutely agitated or violent, medications may be needed (alone or conjunction with restraints or seclusion) when less invasive methods have failed. Patients who present with acute manic or depressive symptoms may require medications to address acute anxiety and insomnia. Definitive treatment of a depressive or manic episode often involves days to weeks of treatment with an antidepressant or mood stabilizer medication.[10] A decision to start a medication for longer-term treatment varies depending on the preferences of each individual hospital. For admitted patients, some inpatient units may prefer to start a medication in the ED in order to begin treatment immediately, whereas other units may prefer to complete their own assessment prior to making medication decisions. For patients being discharged to the community, there is much variability in how often, and in what cases, clinicians will provide prescription medication. Clinicians may be uncomfortable providing prescriptions as they do not want to appear to have established an ongoing treatment relationship or provide medications that an unstable patient may misuse or overdose on. However, clinicians should also consider the risk of sending out a patient who is untreated if immediate follow-up is not available.

Risk Assessment and Disposition

One of the most important aspects of evaluation of patients with mood disorders in the ED is the risk assessment. Risk assessments in the psychiatric ER setting share many commonalities with risk assessments in other settings (outpatient, inpatient); however, there are also some unique aspects.

There are many aspects of risk of harm to self or others that should be considered in the assessment of patients with symptoms of mood disorders. The evaluation should examine not only the level of risk for suicide and homicide, but also the possibility of self-harm, violence toward others, and inability to care for self or for dependents (children for example). Many facilities are adopting standardized assessment tools, such as the Columbia Suicide Severity Rating Scale, to standardize suicide assessment in both ED and primary care settings; however, once the patient arrives in the ED, this tool is an enhancement, rather than a substitute for a thorough clinical interview.

Patients that present with depressive symptoms, especially those with neurovegetative symptoms of depression, may be at risk for inability to care for self. Are they eating meals, drinking enough fluids, and tending to their activities of daily living? Are they taking their medications as prescribed and taking care of their medical problems? These issues can be of importance in cases where patients live alone with few social supports and should also be considered in geriatric cases.

Risk of suicide or self-harm should be considered in patients presenting as depressed or manic. Despite adoption of standardized instruments, prediction of suicide risk is difficult, but an evaluation of suicide risk as part of your emergency evaluation is imperative. As outlined in the APA guidelines for management of patients with depression, the following are known risk factors that elevate a patient's risk of suicide: presence of suicidal ideation, intent, or plans, previous attempts; access to means for suicide (e.g., firearms); presence of severe anxiety, panic attacks, or agitation; presence of psychotic symptoms (in particular, command hallucinations or poor reality testing); substance use; hopelessness; family history of suicide.[5]

In the ED, there are additional risk factors that should be considered and should lead you to strongly consider an inpatient admission. For example, did patients bring themselves in for treatment, or were they brought in against their will? Typically, individuals who are self-referred have greater insight and judgment than those who are brought to the hospital by police or who present as a result of actions of family or friends. Has this patient been seen at your facility before or do you otherwise have reliable records to refer to? Is the patient vague and guarded or forthcoming? Is collateral information available? Although collateral information is helpful in any setting, in the emergency setting such information is often critical. In their guidelines for the assessment of patients with suicidal behavior, the APA points out a number of factors that generally indicate inpatient admission is warranted. These include presentations when a patient is brought in after a suicide attempt or aborted suicide attempt, particularly if the attempt was violent, near-lethal, or premeditated and if precautions were taken to avoid discovery. Patients who have limited family or social supports, do not have an ongoing clinician-patient relationship, or lack access to timely outpatient follow-up are at increased risk. Patient symptoms that suggest inpatient admission are current impulsive behavior, severe agitation, poor judgment, and acute psychosis. Also, for suicidal, homicidal, or severely manic or depressed patients who refuse help or decline treatment, admission should be strongly considered.

In the assessment of patients with mood disorders, particularly symptoms consistent with mania, a thorough assessment of risk of harm to others should be completed as well. The most predictive factor for future violent behavior is past violent behavior, so an attempt to obtain as much data about past violence should be collected; consider past medical records, arrest history, and collateral from family or treatment providers.[6] Other symptoms to consider are agitated behavior, poor reality testing (particularly paranoid delusions), command hallucinations to harm others, and substance use. Mental status changes associated with a reduction in impulse control, such as mania, delirium, or intoxication, are also risk factors. Possible mitigating factors against homicidal behavior include religious beliefs or fear of legal consequences.[8]

The comprehensive risk assessment you complete as part of your psychiatric evaluation can help guide your treatment and disposition planning. The disposition decision will vary depending on the options that you and your patient have available. For example, a hospital in a large urban setting may have an extended observation unit, inpatient unit, outpatient clinic, and mobile crisis team. A smaller hospital in a more rural setting may have an inpatient unit and individual outpatient providers.

A key feature of disposition planning is establishing the most appropriate treatment setting for each patient. The goal of our disposition should be to determine the least restrictive setting that will provide appropriate treatment to the patient while maintaining safety. This decision should be made based on the overall risk assessment of the patient and the acuity of his or her mood disorder—including symptoms' severity as well as the impact these symptoms have on ability to function. Co-occurring psychiatric, substance, or medical conditions, as well as available support systems or treatment providers, should also be considered when deciding on the most appropriate disposition.

Inpatient treatment (voluntary or involuntary) should be considered when the patient poses a serious threat of harm to self or others. As illustrated in Case 2, the patient is at acutely elevated risk of harm to herself and requires inpatient stabilization. Given her worsening depression, suicidal ideation, plan (and recent intent), and family history of suicide, as well as her failure of outpatient treatment, inpatient hospitalization will provider her the intensive treatment she needs while creating a safe environment that will decrease the likelihood of her harming herself should her suicidal thoughts return. Case 4 is another example of a patient with a severity of symptoms that necessitates inpatient treatment. She shows acute manic and psychotic symptoms, has poor insight and judgment, and has been noncompliant with outpatient treatment in the past.

The patient in Case 3 may have benefited from inpatient treatment, but he was not agreeable to a voluntary admission. He did not display imminent danger to self or others, and to ensure the least restrictive treatment setting he was allowed to continue with outpatient treatment. In both Case 1 and Case 3, the patients had involved family members, thus mitigating some of the risk of discharging them to outpatient care. They both also had a history of treatment compliance and showed motivation to continue treatment. In Case 1, although the patient reported some chronic passive thoughts of "not wanting to be alive," he denied active suicidal thoughts, intent, or plan. He also had no history of self-harm and he showed good insight, judgment, and reality testing. Thus, in this case, outpatient treatment was appropriate.

Evaluation and treatment of patients with depression or bipolar disorder in the psychiatric emergency service and the resulting disposition plan have major effects on patients, families, and the community. As discussed here, there are important aspects of the emergency psychiatric assessment to consider, as well as state-by-state legal criteria of which to be aware. The four cases discussed in this chapter highlight some of the common patient presentations seen in psychiatric ERs for those experiencing depressive, manic, or hypomanic symptoms.

Key Clinical Points

- Patients may present to the ED for psychiatric evaluation due to multiple factors, including difficulty accessing care in an outpatient setting.
- Thorough interviews, including obtaining collateral information, are important to assessing risk.
- Patients who do not require hospitalization benefit from immediate access to outpatient care.

REFERENCES

1. http://www.cssrs.columbia.edu/scales_practice_cssrs.htm

2. Way, B., & Banks, S. (2001). Clinical factors related to admission and release decisions in psychiatric emergency services. *Psychiatric Services 52*(2): 214–218.

3. http://www.omh.ny.gov/omhweb/forensic/manual/html/mhl_admissions.htm

4. Thienhaus, O.J., & Piasecki, M. (1998). Assessment of psychiatric patients' risk of violence toward others. *Psychiatric Services 49*(9).

5. American Psychiatric Association. (2010). *Practice guideline for the treatment of patients with major depressive disorder*, 3rd ed. Washington, D.C.: APA.

6. American Psychiatric Association. (2006). *Practice guideline for the psychiatric evaluation of adults*, 2nd ed. Washington, D.C.: APA.

7. Walker, E.R., Cummings, J.R., Hockenberry, J.M., & Druss, B.G. (2015). Insurance status, use of mental health services, and unmet need for mental health care in the United States. *Psychiatric Services 66*(6): 578–584.

8. American Psychiatric Association. (2003). Practice guideline for the assessment and treatment of patients with suicidal behaviors. *American Journal of Psychiatry* 160 (Nov suppl.).

9. Rosenberg, R.C. (1995). Psychological treatments in the psychiatric emergency service. *New Directions for Mental Health Services 67*: 77–85.

10. Ellison, J.M., & Pfaelzer, C. (1995). Emergency pharmacotherapy: The evolving role of medications in the emergency department. *New Directions for Mental Health Services 67*: 87–98.

3

Assessing Suicide Risk in Psychosis

KATHERINE MALOY AND YONA HEETTNER SILVERMAN ■

CASE HISTORY: "I DON'T WANT TO DO IT, I JUST WANT HELP"

Mr. A is a 23-year-old man who immigrated to the United States when he was 4 years old with his parents and three older siblings. He lives with his parents and is sporadically employed at an uncle's business but dropped out of community college a month ago. He presents to the emergency department, escorted by his father, for the chief complaint of "anxiety." The patient initially states to the triage nurse that he is looking for a prescription for Xanax to help with his anxiety. On further interview with father and patient, there is mention that the patient has been talking about suicidal thoughts and that he might be "talking to himself sometimes."

On private interview, patient is evasive and minimizing of his symptoms at first, but eventually he reveals that he has been functioning very poorly for months. He hasn't had a girlfriend in over a year and has lost all of his friends. He dropped out of college and spends his days at home smoking marijuana. He doesn't want to go outside because he feels like people are staring at him and talking about how ugly and skinny he is. His mother made him come to the hospital today because last night he got into a physical fight with his brother when his brother began taunting him for not having a job. He then told his family that he wanted to die. He denies hearing voices but talks about spending his days getting lost in an interior life and has trouble determining the difference between reality and fiction. He adamantly denies any real intent to harm himself and wants to get better so he can be a productive member of his family. He feels he has disappointed his parents. He sleeps most of the day and then is up at night on the internet. He has had no change in appetite but has difficulty concentrating. He states that it is difficult to keep his thoughts organized.

The patient's mother is contacted by phone, as the father states that the mother "knows what is going on." The mother states that the patient has been talking to himself and talking to the family about how there is a "media plot" against him. She is not concerned about him fighting with his brother, stating "boys will be boys," but is concerned about statements he has made about wanting to die. However, she notes that he has only made these statements when family members prod him to get a job or return to school, and he has never attempted to harm himself.

The patient was re-interviewed about his mother's statements and admits to believing that people on television and on the internet are plotting against him. He has some ability to reality-test around this idea. He also now admits to having one overnight stay at another hospital last year, but he states at that time he was using dextromethorphan heavily and was released after intoxication resolved. When pressed, he admits that he had assaulted his girlfriend while "robotripping."

Clinical Pearl

"Robotripping" is a term used to describe the illicit use of Robitussin or other dextromethorphan-containing cough suppressants in order to get high. Dextromethorphan and its metabolites act as an NMDA antagonist and can produce psychotic symptoms as well as serotonin syndrome and urinary retention. This is a particularly toxic drug for patients with an underlying psychotic disorder.[1] Some urine PCP assays will test positive when a patient is using dextromethorphan; however, this is not a reliable method of determining use. Some over-the-counter cough or cold remedies may also contain antihistamines, and so a comorbid anticholinergic delirium may be seen. Psychotic symptoms caused by dextromethorphan use do not typically persist beyond the acute period of intoxication.

Laboratory studies are remarkable only for a urine toxicology positive for THC.

To Admit or Not to Admit?

The patient has a variety of symptoms: anxiety, depressive symptoms, as well as psychosis. He has had a significant decline in his functioning and is now making passive suicidal statements. He is abusing substances. However, he has an involved family who are motivated to get him to treatment, and he himself has some insight that he needs help. He has no history of suicide attempts, and the alleged violence against his brother is not something that the family seems concerned about. If the patient was willing to sign into the hospital, it would be a reasonable to admit him for diagnostic clarification and stabilization. He did not want to admit himself and, given all of his protective factors and ability of his family to help get him into treatment, he was not retained involuntarily for treatment.

Disposition: The patient was provided with psychoeducation about the possible etiologies of his symptoms and a recommended course of treatment. He agreed to start on an antidepressant and a low dose of an antipsychotic medication, and he was referred to immediate follow-up in outpatient clinic, as well as to intake at a program targeting young patients with new onset of psychotic symptoms. The patient and family were happy with this plan. He was advised to start cutting down on his marijuana use, and he stated that he planned to try to stop using altogether.

Follow-up: The patient returned for an initial follow-up visit three days later at the interim crisis service, at which he seemed stable but still exhibited delusional thinking and more paranoia than on his prior evaluation. His father accompanied him to the visit and expressed no safety concerns, and the patient agreed to increase his antipsychotic medication.

On the second follow-up, the patient seemed stable and the father was denying any concerns. He was reluctant to increase his medication any further and admitted he was still using marijuana daily. However, he was still engaged in treatment and denied any active or passive suicidal thoughts since his last visit. He had not yet had his intake at the program for young patients with psychosis, so his treatment in the interim crisis service was continued until ongoing treatment could be established.

Clinical Pearl

While marijuana use is more and more regarded by the general public as benign and by some is considered to be less dangerous than alcohol—hence moves towards legalization—it can be particularly toxic for patients with psychotic disorders. Marijuana contains a mix of pro-psychotic and antipsychotic compounds, and any particular variety or strain may have a different mix, making it very difficult—particularly when obtained illegally—to determine what the effect will be. Heavy marijuana use in young people is a risk factor for development of psychosis, and it can worsen the course of psychotic illness.[2]

Unfortunately, the patient returned to the ED that evening escorted by his mother and older sister. They informed clinicians that he had in fact made a suicide attempt the day before, having gone into a closet and wrapped a cord around his neck, but had removed it on his own. That afternoon after returning from clinic he was found by his younger cousin tying a sheet to a closet rod and fought with family when they attempted to remove it. On interview with the patient on this visit, he was more labile and admitted to an ongoing delusion that he would be forced to kill and eat his family members, and so wanted to kill himself instead as a sacrifice. He still felt compelled to kill himself and stated he would continue to try to kill himself in the hospital. He was admitted to the inpatient unit for stabilization.

DISCUSSION

While psychotic patients provoke a great deal of fear of violence, it is important to recognize that there is in fact a higher risk of patients with schizophrenia killing themselves or attempting suicide than attacking anyone else. Lifetime risk of suicide in patients with schizophrenia is estimated to be up to 10–15%, and it is highest in the years initially following onset of illness and diagnosis, particularly if the individual experienced a lengthy period of untreated psychosis before the diagnosis.[3,4] Comorbid substance use increases the risk of suicide attempts and completed suicide due to multiple factors, including decreasing inhibition and increasing impulsivity, even if criteria for addiction is not met. Suicide risk assessment in psychotic patients is complicated, in that patients may not present as depressed and may not report their thoughts openly. While some patients newly diagnosed with schizophrenia may become suicidal due the enormity of the diagnosis and the frightening changes they are experiencing in their thoughts and ability to function, others may be driven to suicide by the nature of their delusions or in response to command hallucinations. Comorbid depressive symptoms may be associated with suicidal behavior as well,[5,6] although some studies did not find this association.[7] Notably the latter study dealt with patients who were all alive at the time of the review, thus completed suicides were not included in the cohort. Hallucinations may not be directing the patient toward suicide, but may be so intolerable in their intensity or content that the patient feels there is no other escape. Certainly depressed patients conceal their suicidal thoughts as well, but psychotic patients frequently conceal more of the nature of their internal mental state, whether due to fear of being misunderstood or labeled as "crazy" or due to paranoia generated by the illness itself. If you are hearing voices telling you that you can trust no one, or believe—as in this case—that you are forced to engage in atrocities or are being pursued by the entire world, it is quite reasonable to conceal this information, even from people who are trying to help.

Given these complications, assessing suicide risk in psychotic patients requires delving into the nature of the psychotic symptoms themselves to the extent that the patient is willing to reveal them. Gaining trust and rapport requires that the clinician present a neutral and receptive demeanor. It may help to contextualize questions about symptoms or present them as in some way normal. For example, asking a patient, "This is going to sound weird, but are you hearing any voices that no one else hears and that aren't real?" is less likely to elicit a response than "sometimes patients tell me that they hear things that other people can't hear. Or they hear people talking about them. Has that happened to you?" If the patient says yes, then the interviewer can offer supportive statements and delve further. "What is that like for you? What kinds of things do the voices tell you? Do they ever instruct you to do things? Do you feel obligated to follow those instructions? What would happen if you didn't?"

Comorbid substance use is unfortunately very common in psychotic illness and further increases risk of suicide, due to alteration of mood, possible worsening of psychotic symptoms, and disinhibition.

The presence of delusions is not in itself a reliable predictor of suicidality,[8] but certain kinds of delusions and hallucinations seem particularly alienating for patients and thus are more concerning. In addition, individuals who experience psychotic phenomenon are more likely to attempt suicide with an intent to die in response to suicidal ideation than those who are not experiencing symptoms of psychosis.[9] Psychotic symptoms of particular concern in terms of suicide risk include but are not limited to

- Command hallucinations, particularly if the patient feels compelled to act on them or if the commands are distressing in nature. Though many patients who experience command auditory hallucinations will never attempt suicide, patients who have made a previous suicide attempt due to command hallucinations seem to be more likely to listen to them again in the future or to attempt suicide even if they are not experiencing them at the time.[10]
- Delusions that one's body or mind is being invaded or altered in some way by an external force.

- Persecutory delusions about one's closest family or support network. While almost all individuals who experience persecutory delusions will engage in "safety behaviors" to manage the perceived threat, including avoidance of potentially disturbing situations, such as in the case discussed here, these actions are also associated with higher levels of anxiety around the delusions, increased maintenance of the delusions, and possibly even "acting out" in response to the delusions.[11]
- Delusions around the need for personal sacrifice.
- The feeling of "no way out": patients who describe feeling that there is no escape from their situation, their paranoia, or the commands that their hallucinations are giving them. For example, in this case the patient would have rather killed himself than followed through on his belief that he would be compelled to kill his family members.
- Belief in supernatural powers, abilities, or invincibility, which can lead patients to engage in dangerous behaviors, not out of intent to die but failure to recognize danger.

Although suicide can occur in the acute period of psychosis, it can also occur in the aftermath of an episode. Patients who have some dawning realization that their entire world view was predicated on something that does not in fact exist can face a profound existential crisis once their symptoms recede. One study found a connection between insight and depressive symptoms,[12] others have been less conclusive, but on an individual basis, it is easy to imagine the distress one might feel when realizing that one's life has been changed by a serious, chronic condition. Stigma can be self-directed, with patients unable to tolerate the diagnosis and ashamed of their illness. In addition, the negative symptoms of psychotic illness or even the side effects of medications can be quite debilitating. Many of the social stressors associated with a primary psychotic illness, including the loss of employment and alienation from friends and family, can be independent risk factors for suicide and should be considered in the assessment.[13]

While all mental illness carries some stigma, psychotic symptoms and psychotic illness carry the largest burden. It is one thing for a family to say to their friends or relatives that their college-aged child is experiencing some depression and anxiety and undergoing treatment but is expected to return to school. It is quite another to reveal that the child is in fact hallucinating, believes he or she is the devil, or hasn't left the house in weeks due to fear of being targeted by the CIA. Although a depressed relative might be described sympathetically, or even as burdensome or annoying, families may be frankly afraid of their psychotic relative. Families sometimes describe their relative as not seeming like the person they knew or having become someone else. Denial is a very common defense, and families may unconsciously blind themselves to changes in the patient's personality and functioning or attribute it to other causes, such as drug use. Patients may also be unwilling to disclose the frightening things they are experiencing. All of these issues collude to make the issue of "collateral information" tricky in assessing risk. When questioning friends or family about a patient who is suspected of having psychotic symptoms, it is helpful to ask not just about discrete symptoms—that is, if they are seen talking to themselves, express delusional ideas or have periods of disorganized speech or bizarre behavior, or have ever talked about killing themselves—but also to ask about longitudinal changes in personality and function.

Malingering is a common concern in psychiatric ED settings, and certainly there are patients in the emergency setting who will choose to invent psychotic symptoms in order to gain hospitalization, medications, or disability subsidies. Some patients may believe that if they simply say they are hearing voices telling them to kill themselves or someone else, they will automatically get admitted to a hospital or be written for a prescription; moreover, this belief may be based on experience. The astute clinician must engage patients in a detailed interview as well as observing for signs of psychosis that are not reported verbally, such as the patient appearing to actually hallucinate or demonstrate evidence of poor self-care or of negative symptoms. Disorganization of thought process is very difficult to feign for any length of time, but not all patients with psychosis are disorganized, and the presence of a linear thought process is not sufficient to rule out a psychotic process. In general, however, psychosis is not something that is usually readily or easily disclosed, and someone who is eager to share how they are hearing voices is a red flag, particularly when then followed by vague or contradictory answers regarding details of the hallucinations or their content.[14] If malingering is a question, seeking additional information from collateral informants can also help clarify the diagnosis.

Validated screening tools are being used more and more frequently in the emergency setting to aid clinicians in stratifying the risk of patients with suicidal ideation. The Columbia Suicide Severity Rating Scale (CSSRS) is one of these tools, and it has been adopted as the benchmark by the CDC and the FDA.[15] While this tool is currently being used in practice and research to assess suicidality in psychotic patients, there are factors that might increase suicide in risk in a psychotic patient that are not regularly addressed in this screen, such as the presence of psychotic symptoms. The InterSePT Scale for Suicidal Thinking (ISST) is another screening tool that was developed and validated specifically for use in patients with schizophrenia and primary psychotic disorders; it asks questions pertaining to patient's degree of control over their delusions and explores his or her reasons for contemplating an attempt in addition to questions about wishes to die and protective factors. Still, this scale has not been studied as broadly and is not currently widely used in clinical assessments.[16,17]

In this case, once the patient's longitudinal symptoms were clarified during his inpatient admission, he clearly met criteria for schizophrenia but did not meet criteria for a depressive episode, apart from having some depressive symptoms. He had some response to an antipsychotic, and a mood stabilizer was added to combat his irritability. Unfortunately after discharge, he again attempted suicide by taking an overdose of medications and required re-hospitalization. Eventually, he was stabilized on clozapine, which has shown some efficacy in decreasing suicidality in psychotic patients,[18] and was admitted to a highly structured outpatient program, which is not something typically available as a disposition option from an emergency setting. Overall goals of treatment to reduce suicide risk should include reduction of both psychotic and depressive symptoms, alleviation of demoralization and despair if possible, addressing comorbid substance use and providing psychosocial support.[19] Whether this is accomplished as an inpatient or whether sufficient outpatient resources are available will depend on systems of care and available resources in an individual community or hospital system.

Key Clinical Points

- Patients with psychosis have a significant risk of suicide, and assessment of suicide risk should be a part of the emergency evaluation of psychotic patients.
- Clarifying the nature of delusions, hallucinations, and other psychotic experiences, as well as evaluation of comorbid mood symptoms and substance use, can aid in risk assessment and treatment recommendations.
- Collateral information from family and friends can help clarify risk but is not always reliable, whether due to stigma, denial, or lack of understanding of psychiatric illness.
- An open, non-judgmental and calm inquiry can help forge an alliance and elicit information in patients who have difficulty trusting clinicians.
- The early course of psychotic illness is a particularly dangerous time, and the patient may require a high level of support.

REFERENCES

1. Logan B, Yeakel J, Goldfogel G, et al. Dextromethorphan abuse leading to assault, suicide or homicide. *Journal of Forensic Sciences* 2012;57:1388–1394
2. Ferguson D, Horwood LJ, Ridder E. Tests of causal linkages between cannabis use and psychotic symptoms. *Addiction* 2005;3:354–366
3. Pompili M, Serafini G, Innamorati M, et al. Suicide risk assessment in first episode psychosis: A selective review of the current literature. *Schizophrenia Research* 2011;129:1–11
4. Barrett E, Mork E, Faerdan A, et al. The development of insight and its relationship with suicidality over one year follow-up in patients with first episode psychosis. *Schizophrenia Research* 2015;162:97–102.
5. Hawton K, Sutton L, Haw C, et al. Schizophrenia and suicide: A systematic review of risk factors. *British Journal of Psychiatry* 2005;187:9–20.
6. Popovic D, Benabarre A, Crespo M, et al. Risk Factors for suicide in schizophrenia: Systematic review and clinical recommendations. *Acta Psychiatrica Scandinavica* 2014;130:415–417.
7. Harkavay-Friedman J, Restifo K, Malaspina D, et al. Suicidal behavior in schizophrenia: Characteristics of individuals who had and had not attempted suicide. *American Journal of Psychiatry* 1999;156(8):1276–1278.
8. Gunebaum M, Oquendo M, Harkavy-Friedman J, et al. Delusions and suicidality. *American Journal of Psychiatry* 2001;158:742–747.
9. DeVylder J, Lukens E, Link B, et al. Suicidal ideation and suicide attempts among adults with psychotic experiences. *Journal of the American Medical Association Psychiatry* 2015;72:219–225.
10. Harkavy-Friedman J, Kimhy D, Nelson E, et al. Suicide attempts in schizophrenia: The role of command auditory hallucinations for suicide. *Journal of Clinical Psychiatry* 2003;64:8;871–874.
11. Freeman D, Garety P, Kuipers E, et al. Acting on persecutory delusions: The importance of safety seeking. *Behaviour Research and Therapy* 2007;45:88–99.

12. Gallego J, Rachamallu V, Yuen E, et al. Predictors of suicide attempts in 3,322 patients with affective disorders and schizophrenia spectrum disorders. *Psychiatry Research* 2015. Advance online publication.

13. Misdrahi D, Denard S, Swendsen J, Jaussent I. Depression in schizophrenia: The influence of the different dimensions of insight. *Psychiatry Research* 2014;216:12–16.

14. Resnick P. The detection of malingered psychosis. *The psychiatric clinics of North America* 1999;1:159–172.

15. United States Food and Drug Administration, Center for Drug Evaluation and Research. Guidance for Industry Suicidal Ideation and Behavior: Prospective Assessment of Occurrence in Clinical Trials, Draft Guidance. [August 6, 2015]. http://www.fda.gov/downloads/Drugs/. . ./Guidances/UCM225130.pdf. August 2012. Revision I.

16. Lindenmayer JP, Czobor P, Alphs L, et al. The InterSePT scale for suicidal thinking reliability and validity. *Schizophrenia Research* 2003;53:161–170.

17. Ayer D, Jayathilake K, Meltzer H. The InterSePT suicide scale for prediction of imminent suicidal behaviors. *Psychiatry Research* 2008:161:87–96.

18. Hennen J, Baldessarini R. Suicidal risk during treatment with clozapine: A meta-analysis. *Schizophrenia Research* 2005;73:139–145.

19. Kasckow J, Felmet K, Zisook S. Managing suicide risk in patients with schizophrenia. *CNS Drugs* 2011;25:129–143.

4

Assessing Risk of Violence in Psychosis

ABIGAIL L. DAHAN AND JESSICA WOODMAN ■

One of the primary questions to be answered during the course of an emergency psychiatric evaluation is whether patients pose an acute danger to themselves or others, the most basic criteria for involuntary civil psychiatric commitment. The cases presented here illustrate key factors in assessing risk of violence in the patient with psychosis. Assessment of violence risk is a key component of any emergency psychiatric evaluation.

All four of our clinical cases relate to patients with an established history of a primary psychotic disorder, namely schizophrenia. It is now generally accepted that people with schizophrenia are significantly more likely to be violent than other members of the general population, though the overall proportion of societal violence attributable to schizophrenia is very small.[1] The nature and cause of the relationship between schizophrenia and violence has been debated, and research to clarify the relationship has been limited by methodological weaknesses of individual studies and marked design variability that limits comparison between studies.[2] Meta-analyses of the available data suggest specific factors that increase such a risk of violence. In the emergency setting, violence risk assessment is commonly performed as a clinical evaluation, rather than through the use of a standardized violence risk assessment instrument. Both dynamic and static risk factors in the patient's presentation and history contribute to the evaluation of current risk. We focus our discussion on current dynamic clinical symptoms that increase, or decrease, risk for violence, though we discuss static risk factors briefly at the end of this chapter.

CASE 1: SUPERMAN

A 34-year-old homeless man who has a known history of schizoaffective disorder, depressed type, and alcohol abuse was brought to the hospital by ambulance after being observed spitting at strangers in a McDonalds restaurant. He was disheveled, with long matted hair and dirty clothes, and he displayed disorganized thought process. He alluded to being "in movies" and being "Superman." When directly asked why he had been spitting at strangers prior to arrival, he told the doctor that he spat at them after he heard them saying that he was "gay," as he felt this was a derogatory comment and he identifies as heterosexual.

Clinical Pearl

This patient has a known history of psychosis and a known history of alcohol abuse. Many patients with primary psychotic illnesses have comorbid substance use disorders. This patient was aggressive toward strangers prior to presentation. What led to that aggression? Was it a result of his response to psychotic symptoms or due to acute intoxication? The management of this patient will vary significantly based on the answers to these questions. If his aggression was solely due to disinhibition and agitation in the setting of acute intoxication, resolution of acute intoxication, which would happen within hours of arrival to the emergency room, would mitigate his risk of further aggression and violence. If his aggression stemmed from his response to psychotic symptoms, treatment with antipsychotic medication would mitigate his risk of violence. In such patients, risk of violence due to psychosis must be evaluated when the patient is not acutely intoxicated, as intoxication itself will transiently increase risk of violence, but this risk will diminish after metabolism of acute intoxication.

He denied having drunk alcohol in the past day or having used any drugs in the past months. He was found to have a negative blood alcohol level, and urine drug screening was negative for the presence of cocaine, opiates, methadone, benzodiazepines, barbiturates, amphetamines, PCP, or THC.

While in the emergency room, he was initially calm and in good behavioral control and was observed resting on a stretcher. After hours of lying calmly, he abruptly stood up and punched another patient in the face, without provocation. When asked about the incident later, he reported that he had heard the other patient making derogatory comments about him and felt that he had to "defend [his] honor."

Clinical Pearl

Hallucinations in and of themselves do not generally cause someone to behave violently. When assessing an individual with known or suspected psychosis, one must assess for hallucinations. This assessment is based on clinical observation as to whether the patient appears to be actively responding to internal stimuli, has insight into his experience of hallucinations, and what the patient's affect is while responding to hallucinations. If a patient reports hallucinations, then it is necessary to explore the person's subjective emotional response to the hallucinations and the content or the hallucinations. The assessment of hallucinations is not a binary assessment and it is inadequate to indicate *only* whether or not the person is experiencing hallucinations. The assessment does not end with the finding that the person is experiencing hallucinations, but rather begins there.

CASE 2: ARRESTED FOR ASSAULT

A 32-year-old homeless man who has a known history of schizophrenia was brought to the emergency room by a police officer who had just arrested him, for emergency evaluation prior to being arraigned for an alleged crime. He was arrested for allegedly assaulting the police officer, and the officer brought him for evaluation because the patient seemed "crazy." The police officer had observed him standing in a public park and banging rocks together, and when he approached the patient, the patient initially fled and then turned and assaulted the officer.

The patient was born in West Africa and immigrated to the United States with his family as a teenager. When asked regarding the events leading up to his presentation, he told the doctor that a group of five boys he knew as a child had been following him in the United States and tormenting him since he was approximately 18 years old. He described that these young men, whom he named, took on different faces and were disguised as different people. He noted that though these men were black when he knew them as a child, they now appeared as Caucasian. He told the doctor that he was able to recognize them because they had the "same eyes" and "moved the same way." He also stated that one of these men, Edward, had assaulted him earlier on the day of presentation and then had re-appeared to him, this time taking on the appearance of a police officer. He explained that when the police officer approached him, he believed that the officer was Edward and felt that he needed to defend himself.

Clinical Pearl

When assessing a patient for paranoia, it is necessary to ask whether the patient believes anyone to be following them, spying on them, or intending them harm. The patient should be asked whether he modifies his behavior in response to these beliefs. Such behavior modifications can include remaining inside, or leaving the house, leaving curtains drawn, setting up ways to detect whether someone has entered his living quarters when he is not home, changing walking or driving routes, and taking precautions regarding what food is eaten. The patients should also be asked if he knows who is persecuting him and why. He should be asked how he could identify the believed persecutor and what he would do if he had interaction with the believed persecutor. The risk of violence is very different for the patient who reports that he doesn't know how to identify the believed persecutor and would run the other way if he ever believed himself to be in the presence of the believed persecutor than the patient who gives specific examples of how he could identify the persecutor (either as a specific individual or by a sign; e.g., wearing a hat of a certain color) and would want to directly confront the believed persecutor if given the opportunity. "Do you ever feel like you have to defend yourself? How would you defend yourself?" can also be helpful questions.

CASE 3: "LEAVE ME ALONE"

A 28-year-old man who lives with his mother, has a known history of schizophrenia, a known diagnosis of antisocial personality disorder, and an extensive history of incarceration for violent crime, was brought in by ambulance, with police escort, after he assaulted a stranger on the street without apparent provocation. On initial presentation, he was highly agitated and unable to engage with anyone or respond to the direction to remain seated calmly. He appeared to be actively responding to apparent hallucinatory experiences, shouting "just leave me alone." He was given STAT IM medication and placed in behavioral restraints to decrease his acute level of dangerousness due to agitation. He subsequently slept.

Clinical Pearl

Attempts to verbally deescalate and redirect agitated patients should be attempted first, before medications or physical restraints are used. If a patient is unable to be verbally redirected away from agitated and potentially violent behavior, medications can be given to sedate a patient, helping to decrease his acute dangerousness due to agitation. Seclusion and physical restraint should only be used in situations where verbal deescalation and medications alone have failed to decrease the patient's violence.[3]

When he awoke hours later, he was calm and able to engage in an interview. He was preoccupied by and distressed by the belief that his arm appeared "deformed" and repeatedly showed the doctor his arm and described its deformity, which the doctor was not able to see. He described feeling as though someone had been invading his body and trying to control his limbs. He described belief that cameras had been implanted in his eyes and that he was being used as a "tool to see things." He described feeling that the hospital was "setting him up," alluding to a conspiracy between the police, the hospital he was being seen in, and the first hospital he was hospitalized in years previously. He demanded immediate release from the hospital.

Clinical Pearl

Being influenced by an outside force is a thought that can range from an idea to a delusion of reference to the delusional feeling of actually having one's mind or body influenced or controlled by an outside force, which the individual may not feel able to resist. The experience of having ideas or delusions of reference are relatively common among those with psychotic illnesses; these experiences often take the form of feeling that one receives special meaningful messages in what would ordinarily be seen as benign stimuli in the environment (like billboards, newspapers, and radio and TV broadcasts). Less common, but much more frightening, is the delusional belief that someone can control your mind or body. It is imperative to ask regarding such beliefs because patients may not spontaneously divulge them. It is also important to enquire into how much he feels that he can resist such outside influence/control and whether he has ever been in a situation where he was unable to resist such control despite his desire to.

He was admitted involuntarily. During the first three weeks of his hospitalization, he assaulted peers on three occasions without provocation. During his third week of hospitalization, while visiting with his mother and discussing a recent news event that he was telling her was directly related to him (though in fact was clearly unrelated), he suddenly and unexpectedly assaulted his mother.

Clinical Pearl

Patients are sometimes hospitalized because they pose a danger to others. This danger does not disappear once the person is hospitalized. The incidence of violence is much higher on an inpatient psychiatric unit than in the community.[4] Hospitalization mitigates the risk of violence by treatment of the underlying illness as well as by confinement in a secure milieu, which is adequately staffed by trained professionals who are skilled at identifying and intervening when potential for violence escalates or even occurs.

CASE 4: NOT BOTHERED

A 55-year-old chronically homeless man, with a known history of schizophrenia, is brought to the hospital by ambulance after he was observed sitting on the street in freezing weather, wearing only a light shirt and pants, with no coat and no shoes. He was very disheveled, smelled strongly of urine, and had open venous stasis ulcers on three areas of his lower extremities. He sat calmly in the waiting area of the emergency room and was compliant with all requests made of him.

   On interview, he had no spontaneous speech, displayed flat affect, made little eye contact, but did answer direct questions with one- or two-word answers, indicating that he felt "fine," was "hearing voices," was "not bothered" by these voices, had no feelings of being followed or persecuted, did not believe that he was being influenced or controlled by anyone else, and had no thoughts of wanting to harm himself or anyone else. He indicated that he had lived on the street for "a long time," and did not ever stay in homeless shelters because he did not "like" them. He was unable or unwilling to elaborate further as to what he did not like about staying in shelters, merely repeating "no shelters" when asked about his living situation and possible referral to a shelter. He denied having a mental illness, though did tell the doctor that he had been told that he has schizophrenia and indicated that he has been hospitalized "many times" previously, but could not describe why or under what circumstances. He denied having ever made a suicide attempt, having ever been violent with other people, or having ever been incarcerated for more than two days. He did not take any medications. When asked if there was anything he would like or needed help for he stated "no."

Clinical Pearl

This patient has prominent negative symptoms of schizophrenia—alogia, avolition, disregard for personal hygiene, flat affect, social withdrawal—as well as positive symptoms in the form of non-bothersome auditory hallucinations. He is low-risk for harm to others, but his psychosis is clearly impairing his ability to care for himself as evidenced by his remaining on the streets while inadequately protected from the elements and disregarding a need for medical and psychiatric treatment.

DISCUSSION

Epidemiology and Incidence of Violence in Psychosis

The association between psychosis and violence has been observed in multiple studies across different cultural and health care systems. There is strong evidence that both men and women with psychotic illness are at an elevated risk for violence when compared to the general population.

Studies of the association between violence and schizophrenia have looked a prevalence rates in three populations: (1) violent acts in those with schizophrenia, which have generally looked at samples of patients in the mental health system, (2) schizophrenia in individuals who have committed violent acts, which have generally looked at samples of individuals in the criminal justice system, and (3) violence in those with and without schizophrenia in community-based samples, regardless of involvement with the mental health or criminal justice systems.[5] There appear to be two distinct paths to violence among patients with schizophrenia: one for those who have no prior history of violence or criminal behavior and for whom the positive symptoms of schizophrenia appear to be the cause of violent behavior, and one where personality pathology, particularly psychopathy and antisocial traits, appear to predict violence regardless of current psychotic symptomatology. It is very important to distinguish between these two populations, as the treatment modalities used to decrease risk of violence are different for these two populations: for the first group, treatment addresses primarily psychotic symptoms, whereas in the second group, treatment addresses primarily personality pathology.[2]

Large studies and meta-analyses have shown that among samples of patients with schizophrenia involved in community-based mental health treatment, approximately 15-19% had a history of violence.[1, 6] Approximately one-third of patients with first-episode psychosis commit violence with some degree of severity before any contact with mental health services. [7] It is important to understand that although psychosis is a risk factor for violence, the vast majority of patients with psychosis are not violent, thus underscoring the importance of a careful risk assessment for violence during the evaluation of patients with psychosis. It cannot be overstated that the percentage of overall violence committed by those with psychotic illness remains small.

Positive Psychotic Symptoms

Positive symptoms of psychosis have been found to be significant predictive factors of violent acts in psychiatric patients who have no history of violence or psychopathy predating their mental illness. The best-studied of these symptoms are hallucinations of threatening content that evoke a negative affect, command auditory hallucinations, delusional beliefs that there were people seeking to harm them (threat), and delusional beliefs that outside forces were in control of their minds or bodies (control override).[6, 8] The cases discussed in this chapter, Case 1: "Superman," Case 2: "Arrested for Assault," and Case 3: "Leave Me Alone," illustrate patients with these symptoms.

Many patients experience their hallucinations as very real and have little insight into the fact that their experiences are hallucinatory and not reality based. When they hear people making fun of them, threatening them, or egging them on to action, they respond as they would if the experience were real. Such lack of insight rises to a delusional level. Assessment of the patient's level of insight is key. Without the ability for reality testing, learning that others do not share their experience, these patients are more likely to react in response to hallucinations.

Affective response to the hallucinations must also be assessed, since hallucinations that prompt strong emotions of anger and rage are more likely to be associated with violence. In the National Institute of Mental Health Clinical Antipsychotic Trials of Intervention Effectiveness (CATIE), verbal and nonverbal expressions of anger and resentment were found to be significantly associated with increased risk for serious violence.[6]

In addition to the patient's insight and affective response to hallucinations, the content of the hallucination must be assessed. Many hallucinations accompany complex delusions and may increase the feeling of being threatened or persecuted. Less frequently, hallucinations can be commanding in nature. A distinction must be made between harmless and dangerous commands, as well as how often and when the patient is compliant with these commands. Studies have shown significant differences in the level of patient's compliance based on the type of behavior specified by the command, finding higher compliance to relatively benign commands. Familiarity with, or identification of, the hallucinated voice increases the risk of compliance to the command, and these patients should be considered at greater risk than those who cannot identify the voice.[9]

Many studies have suggested that delusional beliefs that there were people seeking to harm them (threat) and delusional beliefs that outside forces were in control of their minds or bodies (control override) were significantly associated with violence.[6,8] A recent study of the rate of violence among patients recently discharged from an inpatient psychiatric hospitalization failed to show a correlation between violence and threat/control override delusions alone, unless associated with anger or impulsivity.[10]

In contrast, prominent negative symptoms of schizophrenia—social withdrawal, isolation, avolition—decrease risk of serious violence.[6]

Intoxication and Substance Use Disorders

There is a high rate of comorbidity between primary psychotic disorders and substance use disorders. Nearly half of all patients with schizophrenia have a lifetime history of having a comorbid substance use disorder.[11] Recent data found approximately four times increased rate of smoking, alcohol use, and recreational drug use among those with severe mental illness as contrasted to the general population.[12] Those with comorbid schizophrenia and substance use disorders have markedly increased rates of violence over those with schizophrenia alone.[13,14]

Greater risk for violence is seen among patients with both substance abuse and medication nonadherence.[15] While causation is difficult to establish, it is seen that this same population has more severe positive symptoms of psychosis than those with schizophrenia alone, which, as already discussed, is a risk factor for violence.[16] There is also a strong association of violence with recent substance misuse, even when patients are not acutely intoxicated at the time of presentation.[17]

Intoxication alone is known to increase rates of violence, independent of psychosis. In addition, alcohol and stimulant intoxication may lead transient psychosis. Intoxication with substances that are undetectable on most routine toxicology screens, such as synthetic cannabinoids and bath salts, are increasingly being seen in emergency departments. These substances have been shown to cause psychosis and have the potential for causing agitation and violence.[18]

Agitation

Agitation can be defined as verbal or motor activity that is inappropriate and often precedes, and therefore must be distinguished from, aggression and violence. Agitation can include impulsiveness, restlessness and pacing, verbal or physical self-abusiveness, uncooperative or demanding behavior, unpredictable anger, and intimidation, which can be understood as warning signs of aggression.[19] The patient in Case 2: "Arrested for Assault" was identified as agitated by police officers when he was observed to be banging rocks together and then fled, both cues of agitation before his assault. The patient in Case 3: "Leave Me Alone" was unable to remain seated in the emergency room to participate in an interview; this was identified and his agitation was managed before it escalated to violence. The patient in Case 4: "Not Bothered" shows no signs of agitation and, as we might predict, was not violent. Early recognition of non-violent agitation is critical; verbal and other non-pharmacological strategies for deescalation should be used immediately to prevent escalation to violence. If a patient continues to be agitated, pharmacological treatment should be offered in an attempt to prevent further agitation and potential violence.

While agitation is often unpredictable, as we see in Case 3 when the patient was visited by his mother and in Case 1, there are situational antecedents that can lead to agitation and violence. These may be less tolerable in psychotic patients than in other mentally ill patients and include unfavorable interactions with staff, including denial of privileges, request to complete or cease a task, or reinforcement of rules or limit setting.[19]

Static Risk Factors

In addition to the patient's current clinical presentation, there are static factors in the patient's history that place the patient at a chronically elevated risk. Static risk factors other than the patient's history of mental illness include demographics, previous history of violent crime or victimization, substance use disorders, and personality disorders. These must be investigated even in the emergency setting. It is known that in general psychiatric populations, violence has been associated with economic hardship, living alone, male gender, and younger age.[2] In addition, a strong association has been shown between being the victim of violence and the risk of committing future violent acts.[1]

Psychopathy and anti-social personality disorder in particular have been found to be reliable and essential predictors of violence in forensic psychiatric populations.[2,6] For those with both antisocial personality disorder and a primary psychotic illness, personality traits have a higher predictive value for risk of violence than psychotic symptoms alone.[2] Both static historical risk factors and current dynamic factors must be included in the assessment of an individual's risk of violence at the present time. Although static risk factors chronically elevate an individual's risk for violence, they are unchangeable and are not likely to be mitigated by hospitalization, whereas current clinical symptoms that place an individual at currently elevated risk for violence can be addressed in the emergency setting and mitigated through acute emergency treatment.

Key Points

- In the emergency room, patients will present with psychiatric illness and comorbidity. These patients are complex and their symptoms require careful and sophisticated assessment.
- There are two distinct paths to violence among patients with schizophrenia: one for those who have no prior history of violence or criminal behavior and for whom the positive symptoms of schizophrenia appear to be the cause of violent behavior, and one where personality pathology, particularly psychopathy and antisocial traits, appear to predict violence regardless of current psychotic symptomatology.
- Positive symptoms associated with increased risk for violence include hallucinations of threatening content that evoke a negative affect, command auditory hallucinations, delusional beliefs that there were people seeking to harm them (threat), and delusional beliefs that outside forces were in control of their minds or bodies (control override).
- Positive symptoms have been shown to have a stronger association with violence than negative symptoms in psychosis.
- Agitation should be identified and deescalated as early as possible to prevent further violence.
- Intoxication is a risk factor for increased violence and a careful substance history as well as drug screen must be performed.
- Psychosis accompanied by an elevated mood or manic symptoms may lead to higher rates of agitation and violence, especially in a confined setting.
- Static risk factors such as diagnosis, demographics, previous history of violent crime or victimization, substance use disorders, and personality disorders should not form the sole basis for violence risk assessment but do contribute to the overall understanding of the patient and his current clinic presentation.

REFERENCES

1. Witt K, Van Dorn R, Fazel S. risk factors for violence in psychosis: Systematic review and meta-regression analysis of 110 studies. *Public Library of Science ONE.* 2013; 8(2):e55942.
2. Bo S, Abu-Akel A, Kongerslev M, et al. Risk factors for violence among patients with schizophrenia. *Journal of Clinical Psychology Review.* 2011; 31:711–726.
3. Holloman GH, Zeller SL. Overview of Project BETA: Best practices in evaluation and treatment of agitation. *Western Journal of Emergency Medicine.* 2012; 13:1–2.

4. Steadman HJ, Mulvey, JP, Monahan, J, et al. Violence by people discharged from acute psychiatric inpatient facilities and by others in the same neighborhoods. *Archives of General Psychiatry.* 1998; 55:393–401.

5. Walsh E, Buchanan A, Fahy T. Violence and schizophrenia: Examining the evidence. *British Journal of Psychiatry.* 2002; 180:490–495.

6. Swanson JW, Swartz MS, Van Dorn RA, Elbogen EB. A national study of violent behavior in persons with schizophrenia. *Archives of General Psychiatry.* 2006; 63:490–499.

7. Large MM, Nielssen O. Violence in first-episode psychosis: A systematic review and meta-analysis. *Schizophrenia Research.* 2011; 125:209–220.

8. Link BG, Stueve A, Phelan J. Psychotic symptoms and violent behaviors: Probing the components of the "threat/control-override" symptoms. *Social Psychiatry and Psychiatric Epidemiology.* 1998; 33 Suppl 1:S55–60.

9. Junginger J. Command hallucinations and the prediction of dangerousness. *Psychiatric Services.* 1995; 46:911–914.

10. Appelbaum PS, Robbins PC, Monahan J. Violence and delusions: Data from the MacArthur violence risk assessment study. *American Journal of Psychiatry.* 2000; 157:566–572.

11. Volkow ND. Substance use disorders in schizophrenia: Clinical implications of co-morbidity. *Schizophrenia Bulletin.* 2009; 35:469–472.

12. Hartz SM, Pato CN, Medeiros H, et al. Comorbidity of severe psychotic disorders with measures of substance use. *JAMA Psychiatry.* 2014; 7:248–254.

13. Soyka M. Substance abuse and dependency as a risk factor for delinquency and violent behavior in patients—how strong is the evidence? *Journal of Clinical Forensic Medicine* 1994; 1:3–7.

14. Dumais A, Potvin S, Joyal C, et al. Schizophrenia and serious violence: A clinical-profile analysis incorporating impulsivity and substance use disorders. *Schizophrenia Research.* 2011; 130:234–237.

15. Swartz MS, Swanson JW, Hiday VA, et al. Violence and severe mental illness: The effects of substance abuse and nonadherence to medication. *American Journal of Psychiatry.*1998; 155:226–231.

16. Large M, Mullin K, Gupta P, et al. Systematic meta-analysis of outcomes associated with psychosis and co-morbid substance use. *Australian and New Zealand Journal of Psychiatry.* 2014; 48:418–432.

17. Scott H, Johnson S, Menezes P, et al. Substance misuse and risk of aggression and offending among the severely mentally ill. *British Journal of Psychiatry.* 1998; 172:345–350.

18. Aoun EG, Christopher PP, Ingraham JW. Emerging drugs of abuse. *Rhode Island Medical Journal.* 2014; 97:41–45.

19. Hankin CS, Bronstone A, Koran LM. Agitation in the inpatient psychiatric setting: A review of clinical presentation, burden and treatment. *Journal of Psychiatric Practice.* 2011; 17:170–185.

5
—

Altered Mental Status and Neurologic Syndromes

JONATHAN HOWARD, MIRIAM TANJA ZINCKE, ANTHONY DARK, AND BEM ATIM ■

CASE 1: LIMBIC ENCEPHALITIS

Case History

Initial Presentation: A 28-year-old Hispanic woman was brought by ambulance and police from her job as a high school teacher. She had left early the day before with a fever and a headache. She showed up for work the next day nonetheless, but appeared confused to her students, making errors with basic math problems. An ambulance was summoned when she attacked one of the school security guards for no apparent reason, biting the guard on her arm. She arrived in the emergency room in handcuffs in a highly agitated state. She was screaming incoherently on arrival with a BP of 200/120, HR of 110. She was given intramuscular injections of haloperidol and lorazepam. When she was stable enough to have her temperature taken, she was found to be febrile to 101.2.

Clinical Pearl

This patient arrived in a highly agitated state, with abnormal vital signs. This presentation is concerning for a substance-induced or medical etiology of her behavior. Monitoring of vital signs, laboratory studies, EKG, toxicology, and careful physical exam are all important initial interventions in this patient. A screening CT scan of the brain could be considered. Acute intoxication or withdrawal would be a leading diagnostic consideration. However, metabolic derangements and other medical problems need to be considered.

Laboratory Studies: Routine laboratory studies were normal and an alcohol level was zero. Urine toxicology was negative for cocaine, barbiturates, opiates, phencyclidine and THC but positive for benzodiazepines, which had been administered on arrival. A CT scan of her head was normal.

Collateral Information: Her family was contacted and they confirmed that she had been acting "oddly" for the past few days and seemed to be forgetting conversations over that time period. They denied all past psychiatric history and knew of no substance use.

Further Observation and Follow-Up: The patient woke overnight several hours later in a calmer state but was unable to recall the events that led to her arrival to the hospital, or even the days prior. She was noted to ask the same questions repeatedly about where she was and how she got to the hospital, and she expressed paranoid thoughts toward the hospital staff whom she felt were trying to harm her. She was unable to consolidate almost any information she was given. She was transferred to the medical service, where she had a seizure several hours later. Routine CSF examination was normal. She was started on anticonvulsants and a-cyclovir pending HSV PCR results from the CSF. The next day, an MRI was obtained (Figure 5.1).

DISCUSSION

The limbic system is a group of structures which govern emotions, memory, olfaction, behavior and helps maintain homeostasis. Although the exact components of the limbic system are not universally recognized, commonly included structures include the amygdala, the hippocampus, the cingulate gyrus, the olfactory cortex, the fornix, the hypothalamus, and the thalamus.[1,2] Limbic encephalitis (LE) is an inflammatory disorder of the limbic system. Afflicted patients develop memory loss, personality changes/psychiatric symptoms, involuntary movements, and seizures. Depending on the etiology, the onset of these symptoms can be quite acute, though they usually develop over several weeks.[3]

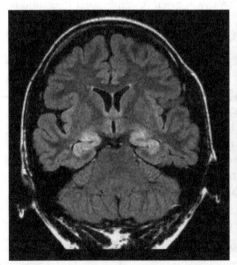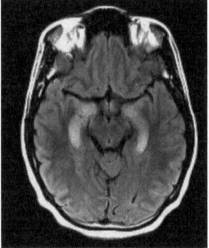

Figure 5.1 Coronal and axial FLAIR images demonstrate symmetrical hyperintensities in the bilateral mesial temporal lobes.

The condition was first described in in 1960 in three cases. Formal criteria were first proposed in 2000 by Gultekin et al. and revised in 2004. The Graus and Saiz criteria are

- Subacute onset (<12 weeks) of seizures, short-term memory loss, confusion, psychiatric symptoms
- Pathologic or radiographic evidence of limbic dysfunction
- Demonstration of a cancer within 5 years of the presentation of symptoms, or development of symptoms in association with a well-characterized paraneoplastic antibody
- Exclusion of other causes of limbic dysfunction

Two major etiologies of LE are recognized: infectious and autoimmune. In cases of infectious LE, viral agents such as herpes simplex are most often implicated. Autoimmune LE can be further divided into paraneoplastic and non-paraneoplastic forms. Paraneoplastic LE, is due to antibody production in association with a tumor. The most commonly implicated antibodies are anti-Hu; anti-Ma2; anti-amphiphysin; anti-CV2/CRMP5; anti-NMDA receptor; and anti-GABA; AMPA; and glycine receptors. The most common associated tumors are small cell lung cancers, thymus, breast, ovaries and testis. In young females, ovarian teratomas (Figure 5.2) are common. LE is often the presenting symptom of the tumor.[4]

Non-paraneoplastic LE is associated with antibodies against voltage-gated potassium channels (Morvan's syndrome), which are ubiquitous in the nervous system but particularly concentrated in the hippocampus.

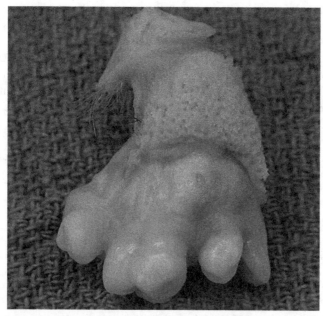

Figure 5.2 An ovarian teratoma showing teeth, developmentally mature skin, and hair. Billie Owens, Ovarian teratoma. 13 June, 2011. CC-ASA 3.0 https://commons. wikimedia.org/wiki/File:Ovarian_teratoma.jpg.

Symptoms of Limbic Encephalitis

- Psychiatric symptoms: Psychiatric symptoms in LE can be incredibly varied, including both paranoid and grandiose delusions, mood disorders, catatonia, and multiple types of hallucinations. Children may present with irritability or hyperactivity as opposed to outright psychosis. In an analysis of 571 patients with anti-NMDAR encephalitis by Dalmau et al., 23 (4%) presented with isolated psychiatric symptoms—5 at disease onset and 18 during relapse. The median age of these 23 patients was 20 years, and 21 were women. In 5 patients, isolated psychiatric symptoms were the only clinical manifestation on initial presentation, without eventual development of neurological symptoms. The time from symptom onset until treatment ranged from 2 to 60 weeks (mean 4 weeks).[5]
- Seizures: May be prolonged and refractory to treatment.
- Autonomic dysfunction: Tachycardia or bradycardia, hypertension, diaphoresis, hyperthermia, hypersalivation, hypertension, bradycardia, hypotension, urinary incontinence. Patients may develop hypoventilation requiring intubation.
- Speech disturbance: Echolalia, decreased verbal output, frank mutism, falsely labeled as aphasia.
- Movement disorders: Orofacial dyskinesias, stereotyped movements of the extremities.

Treatment: There are no randomized-controlled trials to guide treatment for LE, but various combinations of immunotherapy are used, including IVIG, plasmapharesis, steroids, chemotherapy, and monoclonal antibodies such as rituximab.[6] A diligent search for a tumor is required, as removal of the tumor is often curative. Even patients who need prolonged care in the ICU can have surprisingly good outcomes, though relapses remain a possibility.[7,8]

Further Observation and Follow-Up: The patient was started treatment with IVIG for 5 days. She demonstrated significant improvement with her psychotic symptoms, but continued to have great difficulty consolidating information. A paraneoplastic panel was positive for anti-NMDA receptor antibodies and a CT of her chest, abdomen, and pelvis revealed a small, calcified mass consistent with an ovarian teratoma. The mass was surgically removed the next week.

The patient was sent to rehab and at her last follow-up two months after presentation was able to care for her basic needs but could not live independently.

Key Clinical Points

- Limbic encephalitis can mimic almost any psychiatric disorder. Though most cases present with frank neurologic or autonomic symptoms, cases with isolated psychiatric symptoms have been reported.
- It is a treatable disease with a potentially devastating course if untreated and a good outcome if treated.
- It is one of the "do not miss" diagnoses for psychiatrists.

CASE 2: HERPES ENCEPHALITIS

Case History

Initial Presentation: A 29-year-old man was brought to the hospital by his wife for 3 days of altered behavior. She said that he was "not making sense" and was "sleeping all day." She suspected that he had abused "some drug" as he had done so in his teens, but not since their marriage 5 years ago. Beyond this, she denied psychiatric history.

The patient said that he felt "okay," but was confused on exam. He knew that he was at a hospital, but did not know which hospital and could not say how long he had been there or why. He had multiple paraphasic errors in his speech, had trouble following complex commands, and could not name certain objects. He was unable to consolidate basic information, being unable to remember the name of the hospital despite being told repeatedly. He was found to be febrile to 101.2.

Laboratory Studies: Routine laboratory studies were normal and an alcohol level was zero. Urine toxicology was negative for cocaine, barbiturates, opiates, phencyclidine, and THC but positive for benzodiazepines, which had been administered on arrival. A CT scan of his head was obtained (Figure 5.3).

Clinical Pearl

In almost all right-handed people, and about 70% of left-handers, the left hemisphere controls language. For this reason, the left hemisphere is called the dominant hemisphere. Language dysfunction due to a lesion of the dominant hemisphere is termed an aphasia (Table 5.1).

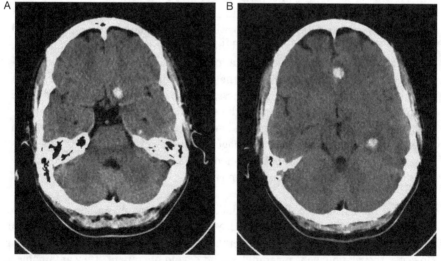

Figure 5.3 Images A and B: Axial CT scans demonstrate small hyperdensities due to hemorrhage in the left temporal and frontal lobes consistent with acute hemorrhage.

Table 5.1 CLASSIFICATION OF APHASIAS

Type of Aphasia	Clinical Manifestations
Broca's (expressive, non-fluent aphasia)	Inability to produce language or repeat phrases, with intact comprehension, patients are well aware of the deficit. Usually associated with weakness
Transcortical motor aphasia	As per Broca's, with intact repetition
Wernicke's (receptive, sensory, fluent aphasia)	Inability understand language or repeat phrases, with intact speech production, speech is nonsensical and patients are not aware of the deficit. Usually not associated with weakness
Transcortical sensory aphasia	As per Wernicke's, with intact repetition
Global aphasia	Patients have a combination of Broca's and Wernicke's aphasia and are essentially mute, due to large lesions in the left hemisphere. Patients have significant weakness
Mixed trancortical aphasia	As per global aphasia, with intact repetition
Anomic aphasia	Trouble with naming objects

Language ability can be broken down into several components that should be tested when evaluating a patient with a suspected language disorder. These include the ability to produce spontaneous speech, the ability to understand speech and follow commands, the ability to repeat, and the ability to name objects. Reading and writing are generally affected to the same degree and in the same pattern as spoken language. Damage to the areas homologous to the language areas, the non-dominant hemisphere produces problems with *prosody*. This refers to the rhythm, pitch, and tone of normal speech.

Different patterns of language difficulties emerge depending on the area of the brain injured and the time course over which the injury occurs. Left-handed patients may have their language abilities represented in both hemispheres, leading to different clinical manifestations of focal injuries compared to right-handed patients. Table 5.1 presents the most commonly encountered types of aphasias. Aphasias, like motor weakness, exist on a clinical spectrum and range from patients with only subtle difficulties naming objects to patients who are utterly unable to produce or understand any language. As patients recovery from their neurological injury, their language deficit may evolve from one type of aphasia to another. For example, as patients with a Broca's aphasia improve, they often develop a transcortical motor aphasia.

Lesions to the left temporal lobe produce a Wernicke's aphasia, also known as a fluent or receptive aphasia. Patients with a Wernicke's aphasia are able to speak "fluently" in that they can put words together, often with relatively proper grammar. However, their language is meaningless and devoid of content. They are unable to name objects or repeat phrases. Patients with a Wernicke's aphasia have disorganized speech, which is often full of *neologisms* and *paraphasic errors*. A *phonemic* or *literal paraphasia* occurs when a patient incorrectly substitutes one word for another similar sounding word, saying "battle" instead of "bottle" for example. A *verbal* or *semantic paraphasia* occurs when a patient incorrectly substitutes one word for another with a similar meaning, saying "head" instead of "brain" for example. Prosody is intact in these patients, as this aspect of language resides in the right hemisphere. Patients are unaware of their own language deficit, and can become frustrated and even paranoid when people do not understand them. Any lesion to the left temporal lobe can produce this constellation of findings. This included ischemic infarction in the distribution of the inferior division of the left middle cerebral artery, hemorrhagic lesions, neoplasms, infections, trauma, dementing illnesses, and demyelination.[9]

At times it can be difficult to distinguish between a patient who is aphasic due to a focal lesion to the left hemisphere versus a patient who has language impairment due to a toxic/metabolic derangement or a primary psychiatric disorder. When a patient's speech is disordered enough that it consists of little more than neologisms, this is sometimes referred to as *jargon aphasia*. This speech pattern often resembles the severe disorganization seen in certain patients with schizophrenia, in which case it is called word salad. It is not uncommon for patients with a Wernicke's aphasia to be brought to psychiatric attention before the neurological nature of their illness is appreciated. This is especially the case as patients with a Wernicke's aphasia often do not have motor impairment, given the distance between Wernicke's area (Figure 5.4) and the primary motor cortex and that they are in different vascular territories.[10]

Further Observation and Follow-Up: Given the concern for herpes encephalitis, the patient was transferred to the medical service. A spinal tape revealed 244 WBC (89%) lymphocytes and 888 RBCs. The patient was started on acyclovir pending the results of the HSV PCR in spinal fluid.

Despite this, the patient continued to deteriorate, becoming progressively more confused and obtunded. Repeat imaging done 3 days after admission showed a marked increase in the size of the frontal and temporal lobe hemorrhages (Figure 5.5).

Further Observation and Follow-Up: Despite the patient's initial worsening, he began to improve after one week of treatment with acyclovir. At the time of discharge to a rehabilitation facility, he had mild word-finding difficulties and problems with consolidation.

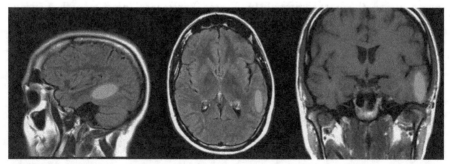

Figure 5.4 Sagittal and axial FLAIR and contrast coronal T1WI demonstrate Wernicke's Area (grey oval).

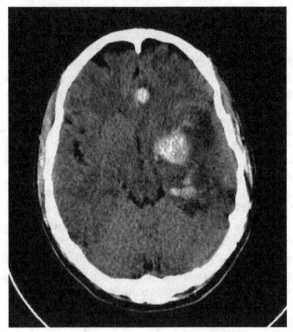

Figure 5.5 Images A: Axial CT scan demonstrates extensive edema with hemorrhage in the left temporal and frontal lobes in a patient with HSV encephalitis.

DISCUSSION

Viral infections can infect the meninges, ependyma, and subarachonoid space (meningitis), the brain parenchyma (enephalitis), the brainstem (rhomboencephalitis), the spinal cord (myelitis), and the nerve roots or dorsal root ganglion of the spinal cord or cranial nerves (radiculitis and ganglionitis).

Viral meningitis, typically presents with headache, fever, neck stiffness, and symptoms of increased intracranial pressure that may be clinically indistinguishable from bacterial meningitis. Over 100 viruses have been implicated in infections of the CNS and in many cases a specific viral agent is not identified. The enteroviruses (echovirus and coxsackievirus) and the arboviruses (West Nile virus, St. Louis encephalitis, and California encephalitis), as well as HIV and herpes simplex virus, are the most commonly implicated. Direct viral infection of the neurons of the brain produces an encephalitis that presents with confusion, psychiatric disturbances, or seizures. Focal neurological deficits may be seen. The most common cause of sporadic encephalitis in the United States is infection with herpes simplex virus I (HSV-1). Infection with HSV-I causes hemorrhagic necrosis of the inferior frontal and temporal lobes, usually asymmetrically. The presumed route of infection is reactivation of latent virus within the trigeminal ganglion, which may explain the predilection of the virus for the frontal and temporal lobes. Patients typically present with an encephalitis of fairly rapid onset, with seizures, headaches, or changes in cognition or personality. Fever is common.[11]

A lumbar puncture will often show evidence of hemorrhage; CSF analysis shows a leukocytosis ranging from 5 to 1000 cells/mm3. Within the first few days, these are primarily monocytes, but over time, there is a lymphocytic predominance. Other characteristic findings include mild elevations of the protein level and o-pening pressure, and a normal or mildly decreased glucose level. The diagnosis can be confirmed by HSV PCR in the CSF. On CT, there is often frank hemorrhage. An EEG will often show periodic lateralizing epileptiform discharges, generalized slowing, or focal temporal lobe spikes.

The illness is treated with acyclovir and should begin as soon as the illness is suspected, as mortality approaches 75% in untreated patients.[12]

Key Clinical Points

- Patients with a lesion of the left temporal lobe may have a Wernicke's aphasia. This speech pattern consists of nonsensical speech, which may be grammatically correct. Patients have no insight into their deficit and often there are no other obvious neurological abnormalities. This speech pattern can be easily confused for the disorganized speech seen in patients with schizophrenia.
- The most common cause of sporadic encephalitis in the United States is infection with herpes simplex virus I (HSV-1). It commonly presents with hemorrhagic lesions of the left frontal and temporal lobes. Because of the high mortality rate, treatment for the illness should begin with acyclovir as soon as it is suspected.[8-13]

CASE 3: A FRONTAL LOBE TUMOR

Case History

Initial Presentation: A 69-year-old man was brought to the hospital after he was found inside a bank, standing for 2 hours trying to use the ATM machine. The patient said that he was unable to remember his code. Emergency services were called after the patient refused to leave the bank. He was taken to the psychiatric emergency room where his wife was contacted. She said that he was healthy, but he had become "paranoid and forgetful" of late. She also said that his legs had started to "buckle" at times and he had fallen several times.

On exam the patient was alert and knew the date, time, and location. However, he was disheveled and seemed indifferent to his surroundings. He had trouble understanding why he was brought to the emergency room and expressed some vague paranoid ideation that the ambulance workers were targeting him. He had poor foot clearance when walking and nearly fell one time.

Clinical Pearl

The differential diagnosis of a subacute change in personality in an older patient is quite large. It includes dementing illnesses, depression masquerading as dementia (pseudodementia), medication-side effects, metabolic abnormalities, vitamin deficiencies, and frontal lobe lesions. A diligent search for any neurological or reversible cause of the patient's symptoms should be undertaken.

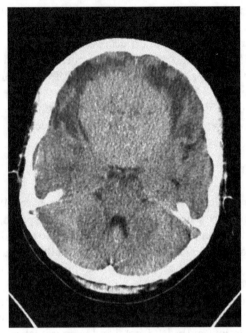

Figure 5.6 NCHCT demonstrates a large, extraaxial mass within the interhemispheric with significant mass effect on the frontal lobes bilaterally and surrounding edema.

Further History: The patient was taken for a CT scan which revealed a large, extraaxial mass within the interhemispheric with significant mass effect on the frontal lobes bilaterally and surrounding edema (Figure 5.6).

Once the CT was obtained, the patient was reexamined and found to have mild weakness in his legs as well as hyperflexia and up-going toes.

Further History: The patient was transferred to the neurosurgical service and placed on intravenous steroids to reduce the edema. An MRI with contrast was obtained (Figure 5.7).

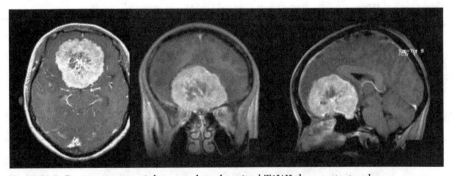

Figure 5.7 Post-contrast axial, coronal, and sagittal T1WI demonstrate a large, enhancing, centrally cystic meningioma arising from the anterior falx cerebri. There is significant mass effect on the frontal lobes bilaterally.

DISCUSSION

The prefrontal cortex (PFC), is the most anterior section of the frontal lobes. Subdivisions of the PFC include the orbitofrontal cortex and the dorsolateral prefrontal cortex.

The PFC is responsible for a crucial set of behaviors known collectively as executive function. This is a set of loosely defined brain functions that includes judgment, abstract reasoning, impulse control, planning, and decision making. Patients with damage to the PFC often show poor judgment in a wide range of situations, cannot navigate social interactions, have difficulty sustaining attention, and are unable to restrain their impulses even when they know they are not acting in their own self-interest.

Not surprisingly, the PFC has been implicated in a wide variety of psychiatric conditions, including depression, schizophrenia, drug-addiction, with attention deficit hyperactivity disorder and antisocial personality disorder.

Perhaps the most famous patient in the history of neurology is Phineas Gage. In 1848, an iron rod destroyed his frontal lobes in a railroad accident. He went from being an industrious, respected individual to someone who was unable to function in society.

Historically, the prefrontal cortex was considered to be a relatively "silent" area of the brain. Indeed striking features of many frontal lobe injuries can be the lack obvious neurological deficits. Patients may have normal motor, sensory, visual, and language abilities. On a superficial basis, many patients with frontal lobe injuries have a "normal" neurological exam. Despite their ability to perform well on neurological and cognitive tests in a controlled environment, patients with frontal lobe injuries are often unable to translate this to real-word decision making, however.

Other features of frontal lobe lesions may include

- Weakness, primarily of the contralateral leg
- Urinary incontinence due to disruption of the micturition inhibition center
- Contralateral gaze deviation if there is involvement of the frontal eye fields
- Primitive reflexes such as the grasp, suck, and snout reflex
- Seizures
- Aphasia for left-sided lesions, neglect for right-sided lesions

An interesting feature of frontal lobe injuries is the great degree of variability in the symptoms displayed by patients. Some may be impulsive, hypersexual, and quick to anger. Other patients may be quiet (termed *akinetic mutism*) and indifferent to their surroundings (termed *abulia*), while others display an inappropriate jocularity, sometimes referred to by the German term *witzelsucht*. Some patients may be frankly paranoid.[13]

These great variations are linked together by behavioral disinhibition, loss of social tact, and poor judgment. The presentation in any individual patient is due to a combination of whether the lesion is to the left, right, or both sides of the brain, the extent of the lesion, the patient's premorbid personality, and the rate at which the lesion develops. Slow-growing lesions, such as meningiomas, can grow to be quite large before coming to clinical attention. In contrast, vascular injuries often lead to instant and often more severe symptoms. The timing of the injury relative to the examination is also crucial, as patients who are initially quite apathetic may eventually become quite disinhibited.[14]

A wide variety of pathologies can affect the frontal lobes, including tumors (both benign and malignant), vascular disease, infections, and trauma. Meningiomas, as seen in this patient, are slow-growing, generally benign tumors that comprise 20% of all primary CNS neoplasms. They are the most common benign, intracranial neoplasm; the most common extraaxial, intracranial neoplasm; and are second overall to gliomas in frequency. They are believed to arise from cells of the arachnoid and they are firmly adherent to the dura and only rarely invade the brain and surrounding bone. They occur most commonly in middle-aged women, and prior irradiation, often for other cancers, is the only known environmental risk factor. They produce symptoms by compressing nervous tissue externally. Clinically, they present with seizures if they come into contact with the cerebral cortex, headaches, and focal neurological findings depending on the location of the tumor. They often grow quite large before they cause clinical symptoms due to their slow rate of growth.[15]

The frontal lobes are often a location for more malignant tumors. Grade IV astrocytomas, glioblastomas, are the most common and most lethal type of astrocytoma, with a median survival of less than one year. They occur most often in people over the age of 50 and are slightly more common in men. They almost always arise in the cerebral hemispheres. Even though the tumor may appear as a discrete mass, neoplastic cells spread along white matter pathways and are invariably spread throughout the brain at the time of diagnosis. Histologically, any tumor with necrosis, vascular proliferation, or pleomorphic cells is automatically termed a gliobastoma.

On imaging, glioblastomas generally appear as heterogenously enhancing masses, with the nonenhancing areas representing areas of necrosis.

The medial prefrontal cortex is supplied by the anterior cerebral artery (ACA). The ACA also supplies the corpus callosum and cingulate gyrus. Infarcts of the ACA produce contralateral weakness and sensory loss primarily of the leg, as this part of the motor homunculus is located within the interhemispheric fissure. Urinary incontinence, to which patients are often indifferent, can be seen due to disruption of the micturition inhibition center. Patients can become disinhibited or abulic. Left-sided lesions may result in a transcortical motor aphasia, while right-sided lesions may produce hemineglect.

The oribitofrontal cortex and anterior temporal lobes are especially vulnerable in acceleration-deceleration injuries, when the brain crashes into and is lacerated by bone at the base of the skull. Contusions that occur directly below the site of impact are referred to as *coup* injuries, while those that are on the opposite side of the skull are called *contracoup*. The surface of the brain is most commonly affected.

Patients with severe hemorrhagic contusions are also always rendered unconscious by the trauma. Patients with damage to the orbitofrontal cortex are frequently disinhibited and demonstrate poor executive function as a result of their injury. Patients with damage to the temporal lobes have difficulty with memory consolidation and develop seizures as a result.

Further Observation and Follow-Up: The patient was transferred to the neurosurgical service where the tumor was resected the following week and the tumor was removed. On follow-up examination, the patient still had personality changes compared to his baseline. His wife said that he was not the same "passionate and engaged" person he used to be. However, he was able to live independently.

Key Clinical Points

- Lesions of the frontal lobes can present exclusively with psychiatric symptoms and patients may have a grossly normal neurological exam.
- There is a wide range of clinical symptoms patients can display with frontal lobe injuries. Patients may become irritable, docile, or inappropriately jocular. This diverse pathology is linked together by disinhibition and loss of executive function and appropriate social behavior.
- A wide variety of pathologies can lead to frontal lobe injuries, including tumors, strokes, and trauma.

CASE 4: BENZODIAZEPINE WITHDRAWAL DELIRIUM

Case History

A 58-year-old woman presents to the emergency room for the third time in 48 hours via ambulance. As per the ambulance driver, she has not been feeling like herself and was brought in from her daughter's home. There was no known medical or psychiatric history. She reported that she is able to function less and less during the last week and therefore moved in with her daughter. She endorsed hearing random sounds of cars in her head and visual hallucinations of birds in the room. She stated she is at home and thought it is year 1932. She was able to state her name. Her vital signs were notable for blood pressure 150/100, heart rate of 98, respiration rate of 16 and temperature of 98.6. Her oxygen saturation was 100% and finger stick was 168. Given that the patient had been medically cleared twice in the past 48 hours, psychiatry was consulted for possible admission.

Clinical Pearl

This patient does not know where she is and is disoriented to time, including year. This is concerning for a medical reason for altered mental status until proven otherwise. The patient requires a physical exam and monitoring of vital signs. Basic laboratory work must be obtained, EKG, as well as a non-contrast head CT.

Physical Exam and Laboratory Studies: The patient had a normal physical exam for the third time in 48 hours. Routine laboratory studies revealed a normal CBC, BMP, LFTs, urine, and negative alcohol level for the third time. The urine toxicology exam was negative for PCP, barbiturates, amphetamines, benzodiazepines, cannabis, cocaine, and opiates. She had a non-contrast head CT that revealed no bleed, space-occupying lesion, or structural abnormality. This CT was the second one done in 48 hours. Mildly elevated blood pressure was thought to be due to hypertension.

Clinical Pearl

This patient is alert and oriented times two and is unable to give a reliable history. Collateral information is key in obtaining information regarding the patient's medical, psychiatric, and substance history. Physicians should also be aware of which substances test positive in urine toxicology and which substances cannot be screened for in the specific test used at each hospital. Neurology could also be consulted for altered mental status.

Psychiatric Evaluation and Collateral Information: The patient was seen and evaluated by a psychiatrist, who also noted the patient to be confused and alert and oriented times two. She thought it is year 1942, when it was actually year 2010. She was unable to provide a reliable history and was unable to provide any collateral phone numbers. She appeared distracted and stated that seagulls are flying around the room. She stated that she could hear motorcycles in the quiet interview room. She also appeared quite anxious and was slightly diaphoretic.

Her daughter's phone number was obtained via chart review. She was called and informed the psychiatrist that the patient has become increasingly confused over the last 72 hours. Before this she was functioning well and working at a local chocolate shop. She also took care of her grandchildren. She was living independently until three days ago. She has no known medical history and has never been diagnosed with hypertension. She has a history of anxiety for which she takes alprazolam. Her psychiatrist passed away in the last month. She has a new psychiatrist, but does not have an intake appointment until six weeks from now. Daughter read the label off the patient's bottle, which stated "Alprazolam 2 mg po four times a day."

Clinical Pearl

This collateral information was of utmost importance in determining the cause for this patient's altered mental status. Given the acute onset, her diagnosis appears to be delirium caused by benzodiazepine withdrawal. She has run out of her alprazolam for at least several days, which could lead to her delirious state and psychosis. Notably benzodiazepines themselves are not detected in standard urine toxicology screenings. Metabolites are detected in 1–30 days depending on the half -life, reactivity, and potency. It is best to contact your specific lab to determine if they can test for the specific drug of choice if in question.[16] Alprazolam is detected as alpha hydroxyalprazolam and can be detected in the urine in up to five days. In this case, the patient probably had not been taking the medication for over five days.[17] Clonazepam and lorazepam often are negative in urine toxicology assays.[18]

Alcohol withdrawal could present in a similar manner, however, the patient has no known history of alcoholism.

Where Should This Patient Be Admitted?

Given this patient's altered mental status and likely withdrawal from alprazolam, she requires an inpatient admission. The question is to which service should the patient actually be admitted. Given that she requires intravenous benzodiazepine medication for withdrawal and needs to be medically monitored, she was admitted to the medical service. The goal was to eliminate withdrawal symptoms but not cause respiratory depression or excessive sedation.[19]

DISCUSSION

Epidemiology and Clinical Features

The sedative-hypnotics and anxiolytics are central nervous system depressants that are widely used in psychiatry, anesthesiology, neurology, and general medicine. Beyond their use in treatment for anxiety and insomnia they are often used to manage seizures, muscle relaxants, and premedication for anesthesia and for detoxification from benzodiazepines themselves or alcohol.[20] From 2005 to 2011 there were approximately one million emergency room visits due to benzodiazepines or in combination with opiates or alcohol; 20% of these emergency room visits led to hospitalization or death in the emergency room. When benzodiazepines were used in combination with alcohol or opiates, this resulted in a 24–55% increase in a serious outcome (hospitalization or death).[21]

Benzodiazepine overdose typically consists of CNS depression with normal vital signs. Most involve a coingestant, which is often alcohol.[22]

Benzodiazepine withdrawal can lead to tremors, anxiety, perceptual disturbances, psychosis, and seizures. It is imperative that this is diagnosed early, as it can be life threatening. Symptoms can begin as early as 24–48 hours or as late as 3 weeks, depending on the half-life of the benzodiazepine.[23]

Evidenced-Based Treatment of Benzodiazepine Withdrawal

Benzodiazepine withdrawal is treated with benzodiazepines with a long half-life. Depending on the severity of the withdrawal, it can be treated with po versus intravenous medication. The goal again is to eliminate the withdrawal without causing respiratory depression or sedation.[19] Other drugs have been tried other than benzodiazepines such as beta-blockers, SSRIs, antihistamines, carbamazepine, and Depakote. None have been found to be as effective as benzodiazepines.[24] In severe benzodiazepine withdrawal patients should be treated in the medical emergency room, medical floor, or ICU, given that their state can be life threatening.

Key Clinical Points

- When patients are not reliable historians, collateral information can be key in diagnosing and treating a patient.
- Laboratory urine toxicology screenings are not always useful, given that substances have different lengths of time that they can be detected. Some benzodiazepines cannot be detected in the urine. Some new substances

of abuse such as spice or bath salts are also not detectable in the standard urine screenings.

- When patients present with altered mental status and psychosis, medical etiology must be ruled prior to assuming a psychiatric cause.
- Patients who present in a delirious state from benzodiazepine or alcohol withdrawal can be better treated on a medical floor where they can be monitored and given intravenous medication. Benzodiazepine/ alcohol withdrawal can be life threatening, so early detection is imperative.

CASE 5: SYPHILLIS

Initial Presentation: A 48-year-old Caucasian male was brought to the emergency room by ambulance workers after his neighbors called 911. The neighbors had heard loud banging against their wall adjoining the patient's apartment and the sound of glass breaking. After repeatedly knocking on the patient's door but obtaining no response, they called 911 out of concern for his safety. New York Police Department documents noted that officers heard what they thought was the sound of the patient banging his head against the inside of the door to his apartment. They also reported that he did not respond to requests for the door to be opened and, as a result, the officers forced entry. They found the patient standing in the middle of a room with superficial abrasions and lacerations to his hands, forearms, and forehead, surrounded by broken glass. He did not respond intelligibly to questions.

On arrival in the emergency room, the patient was agitated and incoherent. He was unable to provide basic information such as his name, address, or current location. He alternately appeared agitated, then quietly internally preoccupied, occasionally muttering a few nonsensical phrases and then drifting off into mumbling and then silence. Due to his agitation, he was given haloperidol and lorazepam intramuscularly to ensure his safety.

His vital signs were notable for blood pressure 156/107 and pulse rate 98.

Clinical Pearl

The patient's disorientation, confusion, and abnormal vital signs highlighted the need to aggressively pursue a potential physical cause for his altered mental state. Physical examination was performed and his vital signs monitored regularly. Routine laboratory studies including basic metabolic profile, complete blood count, thyroid function tests, and syphilis serology were ordered. Urine toxicology was ordered, as intoxication or a withdrawal syndrome were high on the list of differential diagnoses. In light of the patient's physical injuries and the possibility of head trauma, a non-contrast head CT was obtained.

Laboratory Studies: Routine laboratory studies were unremarkable. Hepatic enzymes and complete blood count revealed no markers indicative of heavy alcohol consumption. Blood alcohol level was zero. Thyroid function tests were normal. CT head scan demonstrated no space-occupying lesions, structural abnormalities, or acute changes that may have accounted for the patient's clinical presentation. His vital signs gradually normalized after a period of sedation.

Clinical Pearl

As the patient was unable to provide any meaningful history and initial laboratory investigations were noncontributory, the gathering of collateral information was key to elucidating the patient's psychiatric, medical, and substance use histories. The obtaining of collateral history is of paramount importance in the psychiatric emergency room. Patients who are brought to the emergency room involuntarily frequently minimize or dismiss outright the reasons for their presentation. The patient in this case was unable to provide any history whatsoever.

Collateral Information: Chart review revealed that the patient had previously been seen at the hospital for a minor medical procedure. It was noted that he identified as homosexual. He had nominated his sister as next of kin and provided her telephone number on that occasion. She was contacted and reported that she had frequent communication with her brother, most recently a week before. She reported that he was a highly functioning architect and that he had been in his usual state of good health. She was also able to attest to his having no history of psychiatric illness. She was unaware of his having any significant medical history and stated that to the best of her knowledge, he did not use illicit substances.

Further Investigation and Management: Given the patient's abrupt, marked change in mental status in the absence of any history of psychiatric illness, a neurology consult was requested while the patient was still in the psychiatric emergency room. At the time of that examination, the patient exhibited psychomotor slowing, word finding difficulties, impaired recall and disorganized thought process. He also expressed frankly paranoid beliefs. He was able to articulate that he believed his neighbors wanted his apartment and that he was very angry about this. It was thought that his banging on the wall of his apartment and breaking glass objects may have been the result of this belief. No focal neurological signs were found. A lumbar puncture was performed, which revealed 10 white blood cells (24% lymphocytes), 3 red blood cells, glucose 62, protein 110.9. There was therefore a concern for viral meningitis/encephalitis and intravenous acyclovir was commenced. He was admitted immediately to the neurology service.

In the interim, his serum RPR was found to be reactive (1:64) and TPPA also reactive. Soon thereafter, a VDRL test on his CSF returned reactive (1:16). His presentation was consistent with a diagnosis of neurosyphilis. Acyclovir was discontinued and penicillin G was commenced at 4 million units intravenously Q 4 hourly for a two-week course. He consented to an HIV test, which returned negative.

While admitted to neurology, the patient was followed by the psychiatric consult liaison team. When seen two days after his initial presentation, he was more alert but still somewhat confused and unable to give a clear history of what had occurred. When asked what had led to his admission to the hospital, he stated that he had been thrown out of his apartment by other tenants, as he had refused to sell it. He expressed other delusional beliefs. For example, he believed that tenants in his building entered his apartment while he was asleep at night and stole "personal items." He also reported hearing beeping sounds at night and believed that the sounds were made by his neighbors in order to keep him awake. Significant improvement was noted over his stay. However, he continued to display some memory deficits and paranoid thinking with circumferential thought process. He refused to take any psychotropic medication. After completing his course of penicillin, he was discharged to follow-up with the Neurology Clinic to schedule surveillance lumbar puncture six weeks after his discharge.

DISCUSSION

Epidemiology and Clinical Features

From an historical perspective, neurosyphilis was once a relatively common diagnosis in the differential of neuropsychiatric disorders.[25] The clinical and psychopathological manifestations of neurosyphilis are so wide ranging that they have been called "nonspecific," the "chameleon of psychiatry," and the "great imitator."[26] Syphilitic infection of the central nervous system can occur early or late in the disease and has been associated with psychiatric symptoms generally classified under the various rubrics of personality disorders, psychoses, dementia, mood disorders, mania, and delirium.[27]

The discovery of penicillin during the 1950s resulted in a marked decline in the incidence of syphilis, with historic lows at the end of the 20th century.[28] The disease presented so infrequently that many present-day psychiatrists have never seen a case of neurosyphilis. As a result of its relatively infrequent presentation and nonspecific symptoms and signs, it is not surprising that misdiagnosis has been especially common in the recent past.[27] Since the turn of the 21st century, however, epidemiologists in Europe and the United States have documented a progressive rise in the incidence of infections with syphilis, particularly among men who engage in homosexual activity.[25-29] To add to the potential confusion, presentation in this group of patients is sometimes further complicated by concurrent HIV infection.

Given that neurosyphilis frequently presents with psychiatric symptoms and signs, it is not surprising that a patient's initial presentation is to a psychiatric treatment setting instead of a medical or neurology unit.[27] It has also been suggested that individuals with mental health problems may be at higher risk of acquiring syphilis due to factors such as high-risk sexual activity (for example, in manic patients and those using substances) and patients with impulse control deficits or cognitive impairment.[26] Furthermore, patients with psychiatric illness frequently exhibit impaired insight into their need for care. Stigma associated with psychiatric illness, sexually transmitted disease, and HIV infection often further impede access to care and the initiation of treatment.

Penicillin remains the cornerstone of the treatment of syphilis. If treatment with penicillin is initiated early, it is effective in reversing many of the manifestations of the disease.[27] However, the treatment of the psychiatric manifestations of syphilis is less clear. Various case studies have compared the effectiveness of various antipsychotic agents, but there is no consensus and no clear guidelines have emerged.[27]

Key Clinical Points

- After more than half a century of decline in the rates of infection with syphilis in the United States, there has been an increase in reported cases since the year 2000. The group at particular risk appears to be men who engage in homosexual activity.
- In patients who present with psychiatric symptoms of an acute or subacute onset, especially if focal neurological signs are absent, neurosyphilis should be considered in the differential diagnosis.
- It is of paramount importance to maintain a high index of suspicion and perform screening syphilis serology in suspected cases. If serology proves to be positive, a lumbar puncture should be performed for the examination of CSF.
- The psychiatrist can play a crucial role in the diagnosis of neurosyphilis and initiation of early treatment of the disease, thereby avoiding significant morbidity and mortality in identified cases.

REFERENCES

1. Rajmohan, V., & Mohandas E. (2007). The limbic system. *Indian Journal of Psychiatry, 49*(2), 132–139.
2. Roxo, M. R., Franceschini, P. R., Zubaran, C., Kleber, F. D., & Sander, J. W. (2011). The limbic system conception and its historical evolution. *Scientific World Journal, 11,* 2428–2441. doi: 10.1100/2011/157150. Epub 2011 Dec. 8.
3. Jones, K. C., Benseler, S.M., Moharir, M. (2013). Anti-NMDA receptor encephalitis. *Neuroimaging Clinics of North America, 23*(2):309–320. doi: 10.1016/j.nic.2012.12.009. Epub 2013 Feb 28.
4. Graus, F., Delattre, J., Antoine, J., Dalmau, J., Giometto, B., Grisold, W., . . . Voltz R. (2004). Recommended diagnostic criteria for paraneoplastic neurological syndromes. *Journal of Neurology, Neurosurgery, and Psychiatry, 75,* 1135–1140.
5. Kayser, M. S., Titulaer, M. J., Gresa-Arribas, N., & Dalmau, J. (2013). Frequency and characteristics of isolated psychiatric episodes in anti–N-methyl-d-aspartate receptor encephalitis. *JAMA Neurology, 70,* 1133–1139.
6. Dubey, D., Konikkara, J., Modur, P. N., Agostini, M., Gupta, P., Shu, F., &Vernino, S., (2014). Effectiveness of multimodality treatment for autoimmune limbic epilepsy. *Epileptic Disorders, 16*(4).
7. Pestana, I., Costal, A., Mota, R., Gorgal, R., & Paiva, V. (2014). Paraneoplastic limbic—encephalitis neurologic paraneoplastic syndrome associated with o-varian malignancy—the importance of clinical recognition. *European Journal of Gynaecology and Oncology, 35,* 592–594.
8. Titulaer, M. J., McCracken, L., Gabilondo, I., Armangué, T., Glaser, C., Iizuka T, . . . Dalmau, J. (2013). Treatment and prognostic factors for long-term outcome in patients with anti-NMDA receptor encephalitis: An observational cohort study. *Lancet Neurology, 12*(2), 157–165. doi: 10.1016/S1474-4422(12)70310-1. Epub 2013 Jan 3.

9. Tippett, D. C., Niparko, J. K., Hillis, A. E. (2014). Aphasia: Current concepts in theory and practice. *Journal of Neurology and Translational Neuroscience, 2*(1), 1042.

10. Damasio, A. R. (1992). Aphasia. *New England Journal of Medicine, 326*(8), 531–539.

11. Kennedy, P. G., & Steiner, I. (2013). Recent issues in herpes simplex encephalitis. *Journal of Neurovirology, 19*(4), 346–350. Epub 2013 Jun 18.

12. Safain, M. G., Roguski, M., Kryzanski, J. T., & Weller, S. J. (2014). A review of the combined medical and surgical management in patients with herpes simplex encephalitis. *Clinical Neurology and Neurosurgery, 128*C, 10–16.

13. Alvarez, J. A., & Emory, E. (2006). Executive function and the frontal lobes: A meta-analytic review. *Neuropsychology Review, 16*(1), 17–42.

14. Stuss, D. T., & Levine, B. (2002). Adult clinical neuropsychology: Lessons from studies of the frontal lobes. *Annual Review of Psychology, 53,* 401–433.

15. Mumoli, N., Pulerà, F., Vitale, J., & Camaiti, A. (2013). Frontal lobe syndrome caused by a giant meningioma presenting as depression and bipolar disorder. *Singapore Medical Journal, 54*(8), e158–159.

16. Rainey, P. M. (2011). Laboratory principles. In L. S. Nelson, N. A. Lewin, M. Howland, R. S. Hoffman, L. R. Goldfrank, & N. E. Flomenbaum (Eds.), *Goldfrank's Toxicologic Emergencies,* 9e. Retrieved March 31, 2015 from http://accessemergencymedicine.mhmedical.com.ezproxy.med.nyu.edu/content.aspx?bookid=454&Sectionid=40199370.

17. Mayo Clinic, Mayo Medical Laboratories, Benzodiazepines. Accessed 2/9/2016, http://www.mayomedicallaboratories.com/articles/drug-book/benzodiazepines.html

18. Tenore, P. L. (2010). Advanced urine toxicology testing. *Journal of Addictive Diseases, 29,* 436–448. doi: 10.1080/10550887.2010.509277. http://dx.doi.org/10.1080/10550887.2010.509277

19. Garzone, P. D. (1989). Pharmacokinetics of the newer benzodiazepines. *Clinical Pharmacokinetics* [0312-5963] *16*(6), 337–364. http://link.springer.com/journal/40262.

20. Arnaout, B., & Petrakis, I. (2011). Sedative-hypnotics and anxiolytics bankole A. *Addiction Medicine Science and Practice,* 2011, 511–523.

21. Drug Abuse Warning Network: The DAWN Report. (April 2004). Benzodiazepine. In *Drug-Abuse Related Emergency Department Visits: 1995–2002.* www.oas.samhsa.gov/2k4benzodiazepinesTrends.pdf.

22. Hojer, J., Baehrendtz, S., & Gustafsson, L. (1989). Benzodiazepine poisoning: Experience of 702 admissions to an intensive care unit during a 14 year period. *Journal of Internal Medicine, 226,* 117.

23. Authier, N., Balayssac, D., Sautereau, M., et al. (2009). Benzodiazepine dependence: Focus on withdrawal syndrome. *Annales Pharmaceutiques Françaises, 67,* 408.

24. Denis, C., Fatseas, M., Lavie, E., & Anuriacombe, M. (2006). Pharmacological interventions for benzodiazepine mono-dependence management in outpatient settings. *Cochrane Database of Systemic Reviews,* CD005194.

25. Lair, L., & Naidech, A. M. (2004). Modern neuropsychiatric presentation of neurosyphilis. *Neurology, 63,* 1331–1333.

26. Friedrich, F., Aigner, M., Fearns, N., Friedrich, M. E., Frey R., & Geusau A. (2014). Psychosis in neurosyphilis: Clinical aspects and implications. *Psychopathology, 47,* 3–9.

27. Lin, L. R., Zhang, H. L., Huang, S. J., Zeng, Y. L., Xi, Y., Guo, X. J., Yang, T. C. (2014). Psychiatric manifestations as primary symptom of neurosyphilis among HIV-negative patients. *Journal of Neuropsychiatry and Clinical Neuroscience, 26*(3): 233–240.

28. Centers for Disease Control and Prevention. (2013). *STD surveillance syphilis.* Druid Hills, GA: CDC.

29. Clement, M. E., Okeke, N. L., Hicks, C. B.(2014). Treatment of syphilis: A systematic review. *Journal of the American Medical Association, 312*:1905–1917.

Substance Abuse

Intoxication and Withdrawal

JOE KWON, EMILY DERINGER, AND LUKE ARCHIBALD ■

CASE 1

Case History

Initial Presentation: A 46-year-old man was brought by ambulance after he was found on a street corner causing a disturbance. He was noted to be yelling at passersby and blocking traffic. EMS workers noted that he was argumentative and expressed that he wanted to die. On arrival, the patient had loud, slurred speech and an unsteady gait. When asked about suicide, he responded that he had no reason to live and said, "I can't take it anymore." Attempts to obtain additional history were unsuccessful, as the patient demanded to leave. He started yelling and hitting the wall, and he was given intramuscular haloperidol and placed in wrist and ankle restraints. Vital signs were notable for a mildly elevated blood pressure.

Clinical Pearl

This patient presents with both a behavioral disturbance and vague suicidal ideation, and his lack of cooperation limits the assessment. Given his dysarthria, ataxia, and agitation, suspicion is high for acute alcohol intoxication. Another common finding may be the smell of alcohol on breath. Careful consideration must be given in choosing a medication and dose to manage agitation in the alcohol-intoxicated patient. Unless there are signs of withdrawal, initial avoidance of benzodiazepines is recommended given the risk of respiratory suppression. Therefore, administration of haloperidol alone was chosen, though caution must be exercised as neuroleptics may lower the seizure threshold. Monitoring of vital signs, laboratory studies, EKG, toxicology, and careful physical exam are all important initial interventions in this patient

Laboratory Studies: Routine laboratory studies revealed the following. CBC showed a Hgb 12.5 with an MCV of 96. Serum potassium 3.5 and magnesium 1.5.

Table 6.1 CLINICAL EFFECTS OF ALCOHOL

Blood alcohol level (mg%)	Clinical manifestations
20–99	Loss of muscle coordination, change in mood and personality
100–199	Prolonged reaction time, ataxia, incoordination
200–299	Nausea/vomiting, marked ataxia
300–399	Hypothermia, severe dysarthria, amnesia
400–799	Coma
600–800	Commonly fatal

SOURCE: Ries R, Fiellin D, Miller S Saitz R. The ASAM principles of addiction medicine, 5th ed. Philadelphia: Lippincott Williams & Wilkins, 2014, 43:635–651.

Liver enzymes were mildly elevated (AST 86, ALT 60). Alcohol level was 237 mg/dL (Table 6.1). Urine toxicology which was negative. All other routine labs were within normal limits. He was admitted to emergency observation.

Collateral Information: A review of the chart revealed the patient's brother listed as an emergency contact. The brother reports that the patient has had a "drinking problem" for many years. However, the patient was sober and doing well for a few years until last year, when he lost his job and started drinking again. He said that he has heard his brother has called saying "crazy stuff" when drinking in the past, but he has never known the patient to attempt or talk about suicide when sober.

Further Observation and Follow-Up: The patient was monitored closely overnight. He was sedated following the administration of medication for agitation, and on subsequent reassessments he responded briefly to light touch but repeatedly fell asleep and could not engage in a meaningful discussion. The following morning, he approached a nurse reporting that he was feeling "shaky." Vital signs revealed a pulse 105 and blood pressure 155/95. On exam, the patient was found to be slightly diaphoretic and mildly tremulous. He reported feeling anxious. A dose of chlordiazepoxide 50 mg PO was ordered and administered on a STAT basis.

One hour after receiving chlordiazepoxide, the patient appeared more comfortable. He said that he has been shaky in the past after he stopped drinking and one time he was told he had a seizure, but he does not remember it. He said that he also does not recall all of the events prior to this presentation. He said that he identifies with being an alcoholic, adding, "I can't go on living like this." On further questioning, he said he needs to stop drinking and wants help for his problem, but he has never attempted suicide and has no thoughts of ending his life now. He said that he has had periods of feeling depressed in the past, but these times were always when he could not control his drinking, and his mood improved within a few weeks of sobriety. The last time he was able to stop drinking only after he attended an inpatient rehabilitation program and attended AA. However, he said that he gradually stopped attending meetings, lost contact with his sponsor, and thought that he had control over his problem, eventually leading to relapse. During a discussion of treatment options, he said that he did not know there were medications to treat alcoholism and wanted more information.

Table 6.2 CLINICAL INSTITUTE WITHDRAWAL ASSESSMENT OF ALCOHOL SCALE, REVISED (CIWA-AR)

Patient: —————————— Date: ————————Time: ——— (24 hour clock. midnight = 00:00)

Pulse or heart rate, taken for one minute: ——————— Blood pressure: ——————

NAUSEA AND VOMITING—Ask "Do you feel sick to your stomach? Have you vomited?" Observation.

0 no nausea and no vomiting
1 mild nausea with no vomiting
2
3
4 intermittent nausea with dry heaves
5
6
7 constant nausea, frequent dry heaves and vomiting

TREMOR—Arms extended and fingers spread apart. Observation.

0 no tremor
1 not visible, but can be felt fingertip to fingertip
2
3
4 moderate, with patient's arms extended
5
6
7 severe, even with arms not extended

PAROXYSMAL SWEATS—Observation.

0 no sweat visible
1 barely perceptible sweating, palms moist
2
3
4 beads of sweat obvious on forehead
5
6
7 drenching sweats

TACTILE DISTURBANCES—Ask "Have you any itching, pins and needles sensations, any burning, any numbness, or do you feel bugs crawling on or under your skin?" Observation.

0 none
1 very mild itching, pins and needles, burning or numbness
2 mild itching, pins and needles, burning or numbness
3 moderate itching, pins and needles, burning or numbness
4 moderately severe hallucinations
5 severe hallucinations
6 extremely severe hallucinations
7 continuous hallucinations

AUDITORY DISTURBANCES—Ask "Are you more aware of sounds around you? Are they harsh? Do they frighten you? Are you hearing anything that is disturbing to you? Are you hearing things you know are not there?"

Observation.
0 not present
1 very mild harshness or ability to frighten
2 mild harshness or ability to frighten
3 moderate harshness or ability to frighten
4 moderately severe hallucinations
5 severe hallucinations
6 extremely severe hallucinations
7 continuous hallucinations

VISUAL DISTURBANCES—Ask "Does the light appear to be too bright? Is its color different? Does it hurt your eyes? Are you seeing anything that is disturbing to you? Are you seeing things you know are not there?" Observation.

0 not present
1 very mild sensitivity
2 mild sensitivity
3 moderate sensitivity
4 moderately severe hallucinations
5 severe hallucinations
6 extremely severe hallucinations
7 continuous hallucinations

(continued)

ANXIETY—Ask "Do you feel nervous?" Observation.

0 no anxiety, at ease
1 mildly anxious
2
3
4 moderately anxious, or guarded, so anxiety is inferred
5
6
7 equivalent to acute panic states as seen in severe delirium or acute schizophrenic reactions

AGITATION—Observation

0 normal activity
1 somewhat more than normal activity
2
3
4 moderately fidgety and restless
5
6
7 paces back and forth during most of the interview, or constantly thrashes about

HEADACHE, FULLNESS IN HEAD—Ask "Does your head feel different? Does it feel like there is a band around your head?" Do not rate for dizziness or lightheadedness. Otherwise, rate severity.

0 not present
1 very mild
2 mild
3 moderate
4 moderately severe
5 severe
6 very severe
7 extremely severe

ORIENTATION AND CLOUDING OF SENSORIUM—Ask "What day is this? Where are you? Who am I?"

0 oriented and can do serial additions
1 cannot do serial additions or is uncertain about date
2 disoriented for date by no more than 2 calendar days
3 disoriented for date by more than 2 calendar days
4 disoriented for place/or person

Total **CIWA-Ar** Score _____
Rater's Initials _____
Maximum Possible Score 67

The **CIWA-Ar** is not copyrighted and may be reproduced freely. This assessment for monitoring withdrawal symptoms requires approximately 5 minutes to administer. The maximum score is 67 (see instrument). Patients scoring less than 10 do not usually need additional medication for withdrawal.

Sullivan LT, Sykora K, Schneiderman, L, Naranjo CA, Sellers EM. Assessment of alcohol withdrawal: The revised Clinical Institute Withdrawal Assessment for Alcohol scale (CIWA-Ar). British Journal of Addiction 1989; 84:1353–1357.

To Admit or Not to Admit?

On arrival, the patient's acute intoxication placed him at an increased risk of danger. He expressed vague suicidal ideation and was combative and agitated. He improved rapidly following metabolization of alcohol. However, he remains at high risk for alcohol withdrawal, presenting with a high blood alcohol level and observable signs of withdrawal (tremulousness, tachycardia, hypertension) in addition to a history of complicated withdrawal (seizures). He is appropriate for a medically managed detoxification with consideration for a symptom-triggered therapy or a standing taper of benzodiazepines.[1,2] Evidence indicates that symptom-triggered therapy reduces length of stay and requires lower overall doses of medication.[3] If he did not respond to initial treatment, he requires higher-level monitoring such as an ICU.

The patient denied suicidal ideation once sober and does not appear to require psychiatric hospitalization. If he engaged in any suicidal behavior with potential for lethality or if he continued to express suicidal ideation when not intoxicated, strong consideration should be given for admission to a psychiatric unit. If he requires treatment with parenteral benzodiazepines, he should be maintained on 1:1 observation while on a medical floor. If he is able to tolerate detoxification using oral agents, he may be admitted directly to a psychiatric unit equipped to treat his depressive symptoms and alcohol use disorder.

Disposition: The patient was admitted to a unit specially designated to provide detoxification services from alcohol, sedative-hypnotic drugs, and opioids. Following completion of detox, he should be referred for additional substance abuse treatment. Given his extensive alcohol use and dangerousness when intoxicated, the optimal option is direct transfer to inpatient rehabilitation of at least 28-days duration once medically stabilized.

DISCUSSION

Epidemiology and Clinical Features

A number of studies have assessed the prevalence of alcohol use disorders, though comparison is difficult as they often employ different measures and definitions of addiction. The 2001–2002 National Epidemiologic Survey on Alcohol and Related Conditions (NESARC) using DSM-IV criteria found the 1-year prevalence of alcohol abuse to be 6.9% among men and 2.6% among women. The rates for alcohol dependence were 5.4% for men and 2.3% for women. Lifetime prevalence was 17.8% for alcohol abuse and 12.5% for alcohol dependence.[4] The DSM-5 replaces the diagnoses of abuse and dependence with use disorder. An alcohol use disorder is defined by a cluster of behavioral and physical symptoms, which can include withdrawal, tolerance, and craving. Alcohol and other addictive drug use have high rates in those with co-morbid non-substance psychiatric disorders. Symptoms of depression, anxiety, and insomnia frequently accompany heavy drinking and sometimes precede it.[5]

Alcohol Use Disorders and the Emergency Department

Alcohol is frequently implicated in emergency room visits, whether involving injury, illness, or psychiatric consequences.[6] Patients may present because of a primary problem with alcohol such as intoxication, withdrawal, or seeking help for their addiction. People may also present with another psychiatric condition that is exacerbated by their use of alcohol or other drugs. Individuals may be brought involuntarily to the emergency room in a disorganized state with an unknown diagnosis, where alcohol or other drug intoxication is the suspected etiology.

Unfortunately, people with alcohol use disorders are likely to encounter significant stigma from medical professionals.[7] Population studies have shown that alcohol-dependent individuals, when compared to others suffering from substance-unrelated mental disorders, are less frequently regarded as mentally ill, are held much more responsible for their condition, and provoke more social rejection and more negative emotions.[8] An individual with an alcohol use disorder in the emergency room must be evaluated carefully given significant medical and psychiatric comorbidities.

Evidence-Based Treatment and Disposition

There are several effective options for treating alcohol use disorders. The FDA-approved medications are disulfiram (Antabuse), naltrexone (oral or the long-acting injectable Vivitrol), and acamprosate (Campral). Other medications with promising results include topiramate and gabapentin. While medications for treating alcohol use disorder are not best initiated in the emergency setting, they are underutilized, which may result from a lack of awareness of their availability and effectiveness.

In addition to medication options, several therapeutic modalities have demonstrated efficacy in treating people with alcohol use disorders.[9] These include CBT (cognitive behavioral therapy) for substance abuse, motivational enhancement therapy, and 12-step facilitation (or enhanced referral to Alcoholics Anonymous). Motivational enhancement is designed to focus individuals on reasons for change to resolve ambivalence regarding substance abuse. Alcoholics Anonymous (AA) has several advantages, including low cost, availability, and comparable effectiveness, though some people may decline to go out of a perception that there is a religious requirement. Everyone should be educated that AA does not endorse any particular religion and all references to a higher power are "as one understands him" and the only requirement for membership is a desire to stop drinking.[10]

Patients with an alcohol use disorder should be provided information and referral for additional substance abuse treatment, though brief interventions for individuals with severe substance use disorders in the emergency room are of questionable efficacy.[11] ASAM (American Society of Addiction Medicine) has developed placement criteria which identify six dimensions as the most important in formulating an individualized treatment plan: acute intoxication and/or withdrawal potential; biomedical conditions and complications; emotional, behavioral, or cognitive conditions and complications; readiness to change; relapse, continued use, or continued problem potential; and recovery environment.[12]

Key Clinical Points

- Acute alcohol intoxication is a significant risk factor for violence and suicide.
- If an alcohol-intoxicated patient displays agitation that does not respond to verbal de-escalation, it is preferable to avoid benzodiazepines given risk for respiratory suppression (unless agitation is secondary to alcohol withdrawal).

- Obtaining laboratory studies including an alcohol level are important to evaluate for medical co-morbidities, provide an estimate of expected resolution of intoxication, assess risk for severe withdrawal, and determine if there is co-occurring ingestion or intoxication.
- It is essential to assess for alcohol withdrawal and provide timely intervention.
- A patient presenting with intoxication requires careful reassessment of psychiatric symptoms when no longer intoxicated, given high occurrence of co-morbid substance use and other psychiatric disorder such as mood disorders.
- Despite stigma directed against individuals with substance use disorders in the emergency room, people respond well to a variety of treatments including medication to reduce craving and various therapeutic modalities.

CASE 2

Case History

Initial Presentation: A man whose age is unknown (who appears to be in his 30s) was brought in by ambulance due to behavioral disturbance in public. According to the EMTs, he was shouting at strangers without discernible provocation, and taking threatening postures when anyone gets close to him. A passerby called the police, who in turn called the ambulance. On arrival he is adequately dressed, a bit disheveled, displays psychomotor agitation, and refuses to answer any questions. When approached by the ED clinical staff, he screams at them to keep their distance from him and leave him alone, demanding to be released from the hospital and also complaining about how he has been harassed by the police officers and the EMTs. When further questions were asked regarding his medical history, he became irate and started threatening the staff. Due to the dangerousness of his behavior and lack of effectiveness with verbal and behavioral redirection, he ended up being given a dose of haloperidol and lorazepam by intramuscular injection, as well as going in restraints. After about 20 minutes, the patient fell asleep and the restraints were removed.

Clinical Pearl

The first and the most important concern in cases involving an agitated patient is safety, including that of the patient and the clinical staff. Calm and structured approach is recommended during the first interaction, setting a clear goal that is shared between the patient and the clinician (e.g., telling him that if he can calm himself and cooperate with an evaluation, it would help with his goal of being released).[13] If such method is ineffective, the next step is usage of medications. While any form of restraint, pharmacologic or physical, should be used judiciously and sparingly, it may end up being a better alternative to the patient than potential consequences from further agitation, which may include injuries to himself or even legal problems should he end up assaulting another person in the process.

Further Assessment: Search of his properties produced a photo ID that shows his name and date of birth, which enabled the clinician to look through the electronic medical records for the patient. However, the search did not produce evidence of any past visits. Also a mobile phone was found but the contents were locked and could not be retrieved without the password, and there was no other information about emergency contacts or next of kin. His wallet contained a decent amount of cash along with a few credit cards as well. Vital signs are as follows: Temperature 98.3 degrees Fahrenheit, Pulse 73, BP 123/82, Respiration 12/min, Pulse oximeter 99% on room air.

Laboratory Studies: Blood tests were able to be performed while the patient was sedated. Blood alcohol level was zero. Electrolytes, renal function, and hepatic function tests were within normal limits. WBC count was mildly elevated at 12,600/mcL, and otherwise the results of CBC was unremarkable. Urine tests were not able to be obtained, as the patient is sedated at this time. EKG showed normal sinus rhythm with corrected QT interval (QTc) of 423 msec.

Clinical Pearl

Evaluation of an agitated patient with no available medical history should include vital signs and basic lab tests as well as EKG. In addition to ruling out underlying medical problems that could have caused such behavioral disturbance, these tests can also guide the clinicians in choosing medications that are used for any further agitation that might occur. For example, significant increase in hepatic function tests (such as AST and ALT) would indicate usage of specific sedatives that do not require hepatic oxidation for metabolism, such as lorazepam.[14] Also, prolonged QT interval would indicate avoidance of using antipsychotics, as they may increase the QT prolongation even further, thereby increasing the risk of torsade de pointes, which may lead to sudden death.[15] Lastly, if stimulant intoxication is suspected, there are several medication complications that are possible, such as arrhythmias, seizures, stroke, or myocardial infarction that requires close monitoring that includes vital signs every few hours.[16]

To Admit or Not to Admit?

Perhaps the biggest question for a case such as this is whether his mental status, which was significant for psychomotor agitation, irritability, and hostility that seems to stem from some degree of paranoia, was due to a primary psychotic disorder or substance-induced psychotic disorder. Without available collateral information and longer time for interview and observation, it can be very difficult to distinguish between the two scenarios. Therefore, the appropriate disposition in this case is to admit the patient for further observation, with medications used as needed for symptom management, with the expectation that his condition would improve after the effects of the substance (or multiple substances) wear off.

Reassessment: The patient stayed asleep for the next 6 hours. When he awoke he was irritable but lethargic, and went back to sleep readily. Two hours later he was he awoke again and managed to eat a little bit of the meal provided for him. He used the restroom and complied with providing a urine sample. He was still rather lethargic, somewhat irritable when approached but did not appear paranoid anymore. Urine toxicology was positive for cocaine and benzodiazepine, and negative for opiate, amphetamine, cannabis, and phencyclidine. Repeated vital signs are as follows: Temperature 97.9 degrees Fahrenheit, Pulse 68, BP 112/70, Respiration 14/min, Pulse oximeter 98% on room air.

Clinical Pearl

While urine toxicology result confirms recent cocaine use, this does not necessarily mean that the presentation is solely due to cocaine intoxication, since the metabolite of cocaine detected in urine, benzoylecgonine, can be detected for two to 3 days after last use.[17] Furthermore, it does not rule out concomitant use of other substances that may cause agitation that are not yet routinely detected in toxicology, such as synthetic cannabinoids (such as "Spice" and "K2"), methylenedioxypyrovalerone (MDPV or "Bath Salts"), or MDMA (known as "Ecstasy" or "Molly").[18,19,20] Furthermore, the toxicology result alone cannot rule out presence of primary psychotic disorder that may have been acutely exacerbated by substance use. Positive detection of benzodiazepine could suggest agitation due to withdrawal, or detection of benzodiazepine that was given in the ED for agitation hours earlier. When you consider the patient's overall condition at this point, particularly the presence lethargy and irritability along with absence of paranoia after several hours, the most likely diagnosis is cocaine-induced psychotic disorder.

Disposition: After the patient spent another 8 hours on observation, he was able to be awakened easily and now cooperative with an interview despite still being somewhat lethargic. The patient confirmed use of cocaine a few hours prior to presentation. He remembered feeling very anxious around others at that time, feeling unsafe around them as if they might hurt him. He did not recall any auditory, visual, or tactile hallucinations at the time. He denied use of any other substances. He stated that his mood was "tired," with constricted affect, with no suicidal or violent ideation toward others. When asked about his level of use, he denied that he uses any drugs on a regular basis, and did not see it as a problem for him. While he was appropriately concerned about the events that transpired that led to his presentation, he refused to any referrals to substance abuse treatment resources. He was discharged from the hospital as he requested.

DISCUSSION

There are several types of substance that can lead to agitation. The first that may come to the minds of most clinicians is stimulant, which includes substances such as cocaine, amphetamines, and newly emerging substances such as MDPV. As the name suggests, stimulants may cause agitation and irritability as well as other physical signs, such as tachycardia, hypertension, bruxism, to name a few.[16,19] Symptoms of psychosis may also occur alongside, most often paranoia, and less frequently hallucinations that tend to have paranoid themes.[21] However, it is important to note that other substances may first cause psychotic symptoms, which can in turn lead to agitation and impulsive behavior. These substances may include phencyclidine (PCP), which is unique in mimicking not just the positive symptoms of schizophrenia (e.g., delusions and hallucinations) but also the negative symptoms of schizophrenia (e.g., alogia, flat affect).[21] Certain strains of cannabis may induce more psychotic symptoms than others, depending on the ratio of THC and cannabidiol, latter of which actually has antipsychotic effect.[22] Synthetic cannabinoids, on the other hand, can act as agonist at the cannabinoid receptors, which may induce psychotic symptoms as THC can, but lack cannabidiol and its antipsychotic effect and thus may cause substantial degree of psychosis.[18] MDMA intoxication can have effects that are like stimulants as well as a sense of empathy and bond with others.[23] While it is typically classified as a depressant, alcohol intoxication may lead to significantly impaired impulse control. Moreover, presence of ethanol in the body with cocaine leads to formation of a new compound, cocaethylene, is produced that is associated with higher level of violence and cardiotoxicity.[24] It is important also to consider complicated withdrawal in the differential diagnosis of agitation, particularly from alcohol, sedative-hypnotics, and opioids. It is unlikely that opioid withdrawal will lead to psychotic symptoms, but withdrawal from either alcohol or sedative-hypnotics may cause hallucination and disorientation.[25,26] Finally, it is important to remember that one cannot simply rule out a primary psychiatric disorder just because substance intoxication or withdrawal is confirmed. Therefore, the most prudent course of action in dealing with such patients is to observe them until the effects of the substances wear off, and then see how the patient's mental status looks like at that point.

Key Clinical Points

- Safety is the first and most important concern in treatment of agitated patients. Verbal and behavioral redirection should be attempted prior to more restrictive methods, such as chemical and physical restraints.
- Medical evaluation and monitoring is essential if a patient is to be observed in the ED, serving the purposes of finding the correct cause of the behavioral disturbance as well as detecting any potential complications of substance intoxication or withdrawal.
- While certain medications are relied upon heavily for purposes of treating agitation, the regimen may need to be changed based on the results of lab tests and EKG as well as potential adverse effects.
- The patient should be reassessed after the effects of substances dissipate, as withdrawal from substances such as stimulants may cause depression and suicidal thoughts. Also, the reassessment can also help detect any underlying psychiatric disorder, which may affect the subsequent disposition.

CASE 3

Case History

Initial Presentation: A 27-year-old woman is found unresponsive at home, and brought into the emergency room by EMS. En route to the emergency room, the EMTs noted pinpoint pupils, shallow respirations of 6 per minute, and multiple "track marks" on her arms. They empirically gave her intramuscular naloxone prior to arrival to the emergency room, and by the time they pulled into the ambulance bay, the patient was highly agitated, yelling, threatening the EMS workers, and attempting to jump out of the stretcher. She required multiple hospital staff members to restrain her for her safety, and she continued to scream as she was wheeled into the emergency department.

Clinical Pearl

The patient's initial presentation, including non-responsiveness, miosis, and respiratory depression were all consistent with opiate overdose. The sedation and respiratory depression are due to the effects of opiates on the mu-opioid receptors in the central nervous system (CNS).[27] The intramuscular naloxone, an opioid antagonist, quickly reversed the effects of the opiates in the patient's system, precipitating withdrawal and leading to her agitation. While naltrexone can be given intravenously (doses of 0.4–0.8 mg are usually sufficient to quickly reverse the respiratory depression and sedation), it can often be given more quickly via the intramuscular route in the field. Additionally, since 1996 in the United States, opioid overdose prevention programs have been developed to train members of the community to recognize the symptoms of opioid overdose and to administer intranasal formulations of naloxone ("Narcan kits"), with distribution of these kits to high-risk individuals and their families intended to attempt to reduce the number of deaths by accidental overdose.[28] A 2009 randomized controlled trial by Kerr et al. demonstrated similar efficacy of intranasal and intramuscular routes of administration.[29]

In the emergency department, the patient was placed in wrist and ankle restraints for safety, and was given 5 mg of intramuscular haloperidol due to her continued agitation. Co-administration of a benzodiazepine was avoided due to the risk of respiratory suppression when combined with opioids. When she was sufficiently calm, blood was obtained for laboratory studies, and a urine sample was collected.

Laboratory Studies: Serum electrolytes and complete blood count were within normal limits, hepatic enzymes were mildly elevated to twice the upper limit of normal, alcohol level was 150 mg/dL. Serum bHCG was negative. Urine toxicology was positive for opiates and methadone, and negative for cocaine, cannabis, benzodiazepines, amphetamines, and phencyclidine. Electrocardiogram showed normal sinus rhythm, heart rate of 70, with a QTc of 495.

Forty-five minutes after her arrival to the emergency department, the patient's pulse-oximeter alarm sounded, and she was noted to again be non-responsive, with breathing again shallow, at 4 breaths per minute.

Clinical Pearl

Naloxone, which has a quick onset of action, also has a short half-life of approximately one hour. Multiple doses may be required, particularly when a patient has used a long-acting opioid (ex. Methadone) or an especially potent opioid (ex. Fentanyl). Individuals should be observed in the emergency setting for several hours to ensure that there is not a recurrence of symptoms.

Methadone can prolong the QTc, so caution should be used when administering other medications, including many of the second-generation antipsychotics that also are associated with QTc prolongation, in patients who are prescribed, or illicitly use, methadone.[30]

Collateral Information: The patient's parents are contacted, and report that she has a long history of addiction to both prescription opioids and heroin, which led to her dropping out of the college and being kicked out of their house due to stealing money from them in the past. She had been on maintenance methadone for 2 years, but that she had recently attended an inpatient detoxification and rehabilitation program and had expressed a desire to be "drug-free" without any methadone or buprenorphine maintenance. They were unaware, though not shocked, that she had relapsed on drugs.

Clinical Pearl

Relapse rates following inpatient treatment can be as high as 60%.[31] For individuals not on agonist therapy, following inpatient treatment, their opiate tolerance is significantly lower, and they are at much higher risk of potentially fatal overdose, as in this case.

Further Observation and Follow-Up: The patient received two additional doses of intravenous naloxone, and she was monitored closely in the emergency setting for 6 hours. Her vital signs remained stable, and while she did not display any more significant agitation as she had on arrival, she complained of muscle pain and nausea, as well as anxiety. She became tearful, and was overheard by a nurse saying she felt so horrible she wanted to die, which led the emergency team to consult the on-call psychiatrist.

Clinical Pearl

Management of precipitated opiate withdrawal, as in this case, should be supportive, and administration of opioids is contraindicated due to the short half-life of the naltrexone, and the potential for overdose.[32]

The patient met with the psychiatrist, who initially recommended she be clonidine 0.1 mg, ibuprofen, and ondansetron IM to help with her withdrawal symptoms. Once she was feeling physically better, she explained to the psychiatrist that while she had tried hard to maintain abstinence following her discharge from inpatient rehab 2 weeks ago, she had no longer been able to resist her cravings and had relapsed first on methadone she bought on the street 4 days ago and then IV heroin the day prior to admission. She describes tearfully that she wants to be free of heroin, and wonders if she should return to a methadone treatment program, though she also laments how difficult it had been to get to the clinic each day since she has also been trying to work at the time. She said that she had maintained abstinence from heroin and other illicit substances during the 2 years that she was enrolled in the methadone program, but she had wanted to detox from methadone due, in part, to pressure she felt from some of her friends at Narcotics Anonymous (N.A.) that she should be "drug free." However, when she stopped treatment in the methadone program, she soon relapsed, using up to 15 bags of heroin intravenously daily, until she entered the inpatient treatment program the month before. In total, she has attended four inpatient rehab programs (all of which were 28-day programs) and two outpatient programs; her longest period of abstinence from heroin since she started using at age 19 was the 2 years she was in the methadone program. At other times, without methadone maintenance, she has not been able to maintain more than 2 months of sobriety at a time. She has never had an overdose leading to emergency presentation before. She denies recent symptoms of depression prior to her relapse, stating that she was feeling "good" when she left inpatient treatment, was enjoying being clean and sober, and was eating and sleeping well. She denied any prior history of manic or psychotic symptoms, denied prior psychiatric treatment other than for substance abuse, and denied any history of suicide attempts or violence. She reported one prior arrest for a drug possession charge for which she did not have to serve time in jail. Regarding the statement overheard by the nurse about wanting to die, the patient said that she felt so physically horrible at that moment, she said that to try to get someone to pay attention to her distress, but she denied any suicidal plan or intent. She said multiple times that she was lucky that the overdose had not killed her, and that she thought she had calculated a safe amount of heroin to take to get "high" without overdosing, but she had not realized how low her tolerance had become. The psychiatrist also spoke with the patient's parents, recently arrived at their daughter's bedside, who confirmed that she had no known psychiatric history other than substance abuse, and that she had no history, to their knowledge, of suicide attempts.

To Admit or Not to Admit?

The consulting psychiatrist felt that the patient did not have evidence of psychiatric symptoms or a level of risk of intentional harm to self and others that necessitated in inpatient level of psychiatric care. However, given the patient's history of multiple attempts at inpatient treatment, with frequent relapses when off of methadone maintenance, the psychiatrist, the patient, and her parents agreed that she should reenter an inpatient treatment program and return to methadone maintenance.

Clinical Pearl

The American Society of Addiction Medicine (ASAM) has published placement criteria to help clinicians, families, and patients determine the appropriate level of care for an individual. These criteria include assessment of the patient's current level of intoxication and withdrawal risk, medical and psychiatric comorbidities, their readiness to change, their history or potential for relapse, and the supports available in their home environment.[33] See previous section about alcohol use disorder for further information about the ASAM criteria.

In the emergency or inpatient setting, methadone may be given to manage opioid withdrawal. Generally a dose of 10–15 mg is sufficient to manage most of the withdrawal symptoms; higher doses carry risk of respiratory suppression. Methadone maintenance treatment cannot be initiated outside of a federally licensed program. If a patient presents to the emergency department and states that they are in a methadone program, the MD or RN should contact the program and document the amount and date of the last methadone dose prior to the MD prescribing a dose in the emergency or inpatient setting. If the patient has missed more than 1 day of methadone treatment, the dose should be reduced to avoid risk of overdose.

Disposition: The patient, her parents, and the psychiatrist talked at length about treatment options, and the emergency department social worker met with them as well to provide referrals. Somewhat reluctantly, the patient agreed to enter a therapeutic community for long-term residential treatment. They were all pleased to find a therapeutic community that was also a federally licensed methadone treatment program. The program offered the patient an appointment for admission the following morning, and the patient and her parents agreed she would stay with her parents that night and they would take her to the program in the morning.

DISCUSSION

The American Psychiatric Association, in the DSM-5, defines opioid use disorder as a pattern of use causing significant impairment or distress, with at least two of the symptoms present for the disorder. Symptoms include escalating use, repeated unsuccessful attempts to cut back, significant time devoted to obtaining and/or using opioids, cravings, failure to meet obligations, persistent use despite consequences, recurrent use in hazardous situations, continued use despite worsening health consequences of use, tolerance, and withdrawal. Opioid use disorders are classified as mild (2–3 symptoms), moderate (4–5 symptoms) or severe (6+ symptoms).[5]

This case highlights a young woman with a severe level of opioid use disorder (defined by demonstrating at least 6 of the symptoms described earlier). She had often used in greater amounts than intended, had made repeated attempts to control her use, had use which impaired her ability to fulfill obligations (and had led to her dropping out of college and losing several jobs), and had developed tolerance as well as withdrawal symptoms in the past. The case also highlights considerations that can be made for treatment, including pharmacotherapy and psychosocial treatment options.

Epidemiology and Clinical Features

Opioid use disorders include use of both illicit substances (e.g., heroin), and prescription medications that are either prescribed or obtained through illicit means (e.g., oxycodone, methadone). The National Survey on Drug Use and Health in 2013 estimated that in the United States, there are 2.1 million Americans addicted to prescription opiates (though this number may be inaccurately low, as the survey only asked about agents that were not prescribed to the user) and 467,000 heroin users.[34] A recent systematic review explored determinants of the dramatic increase in drug overdose deaths in the United States in recent years, which included a more than four-fold increase in the amount of these deaths in which prescription opiates were involved from 1999–2010, with a similar increase in sales of prescription opiates in healthcare settings during those years.[35] This study also highlighted that "prescription of more potent opioids, particularly methadone and long-acting forms of oxycodone, has increased most rapidly, with associated increases in mortality."[35] Historically, dramatic increases in opioid prescriptions followed the 1995 introduction of oxycontin on the market, and a significant pharma-sponsored campaign to increase the long-term use of opioids for non-cancer pain, and was linked to the development of the "Pain Is the Fifth Vital Sign" campaign started at the 1995 annual meeting of the American Pain Society.[34] Between 1997 and 2011, the number of individuals seeking treatment for addictions to prescription opiates increased by 900%.[34]

Given the dramatic increase in opioid overdoses, the Centers for Disease Control added in 2014 opioid overdose prevention to its list of top-five public health challenges.[34] In their review of the public health crisis caused by the increase in prescription opioids, Kolodny et al. state, "according to the federal government's National Survey on Drug Use and Health (NSDUH), 4 out of 5 current heroin users report that their opioid use began with OPRs [opioid pain relievers]. Many of these individuals appear to be switching to heroin after becoming addicted to OPRs because heroin is less expensive on the black market."[3]

Evidence-Based Treatment and Disposition

Treatment of opiate use disorders includes both the emergency management of opiate overdose, in which the opiate receptor antagonist naloxone, along with supportive measures, is the standard of care. For individuals with opiate use disorders, treatment options can include residential, inpatient or outpatient levels of care (see earlier description of the ASAM placement criteria). Additional supports in the community can include twelve-step programs, including Narcotics Anonymous. For many individuals pharmacotherapy is indicated. There are three main options: agonist therapy with methadone, partial-agonist therapy with buprenorphine (usually in combination with naloxone, which is included in the tablet or sublingual strip, and has limited oral bioavailability, but is included in the formulation to prevent injection of the medication) and agonist therapy with naltrexone (which can be prescribed orally, or in a long-acting intramuscular injection). Therapy with methadone or buprenorphine is aimed primarily at preventing opiate cravings, whereas naltrexone prevents the individual from experiencing the "high" if they do use opiates. Methadone maintenance therapy can only be administered through a federally licensed program, in which guidelines are in place regulating frequency of patient visits (individuals all start with at least a 6-day per week "pick-up" schedule). Buprenorphine can be prescribed by individual physicians in an office setting if the physician has completed the required training needed to receive the required prescription waiver.

In addition, specific public health measures are aimed at reducing the mortality of opiate overdose, including public education campaigns and the distribution of naloxone kits in the community. Efforts to stem the flood of prescription opiates in the community include education of physicians, policies that reduce prescriptions provided in emergency settings, and prescription monitoring programs in some states, which help reduce "doctor-shopping" for prescriptions.[34]

Key Clinical Points

- Symptoms of opioid overdose include unresponsiveness, respiratory depression, and pinpoint pupils. Symptoms respond quickly to naloxone (which can be given intranasally in the community, intramuscularly en route to the hospital, and intravenously in the hospital).
- Naloxone administration can precipitate acute withdrawal, which is very uncomfortable for the patient and may lead to agitation. However, clinicians should also bear in mind that the duration of action of naloxone is short, and multiple doses may be required, particularly if the patient has used long-acting opioids like methadone.
- Methadone at 10–15 mg can safely treat opioid withdrawal symptoms in the emergency setting, but doses higher than that carry the risk of respiratory suppression (unless there is confirmation from the patient's methadone program of their maintenance dose).
- Initiation of methadone maintenance treatment cannot be done outside a federally licensed program.
- Other evidence-based pharmacologic treatments for opioid use disorders include buprenorphine and intramuscular naltrexone.

REFERENCES

1. Ries R, Fiellin D, Miller S, Saitz R. The ASAM principles of addiction medicine, 5th ed. Philadelphia: Lippincott Williams & Wilkins, 2014, 43:635–651.
2. Sullivan JT, Sykora K, Schneiderman J, Naranjo CA, Sellers EM. Assessment of alcohol withdrawal: The revised Clinical Institute Withdrawal Assessment for Alcohol scale (CIWA-Ar). Brit J Addict 1989; 84:1353–1357.
3. Saitz R, Mayo-Smith MF, Roberts MS, et al. Individualized treatment for alcohol withdrawal: A randomized double blind controlled trial. JAMA 1994; 272:519–523.
4. Hasin DS, Stinson FS, Ogburn E, et al. Prevalence, correlates, disability, and comorbidity of DSM-IV alcohol abuse and dependence in the United States: Results from the National Epidemiologic Survey on alcohol and related conditions. Arch Gen Psychiatry 2007; 64(7):830–842.
5. American Psychiatric Association. *Diagnostic and statistical manual of mental disorders: DSM-5.* Washington, D.C: American Psychiatric Association, 2013.
6. Rockett IRH, Putnam SL, Jia H, et al. Declared and undeclared substance use among emergency department patients: a population-based study. *Addiction* 2006; 101:706–712.

7. Van Boekel LC, Brouwers EP, Van Weeghel J, Garretsen HF. Healthcare professionals' regard towards working with patients with substance use disorders: Comparison of primary care, general psychiatry and specialist addiction services. Drug Alcohol Depend Jan 1 2014; 134:92–98.

8. Schomerus G, Lucht M, Holzinger A, Matschinger H, Carta MG, Angermeyer MC. The stigma of alcohol dependence compared with other mental disorders: A review of population studies. Alcohol 2011; 46:105–112.

9. Project MATCH Research Group. Matching alcoholism treatments to client heterogeneity: Project MATCH posttreatment drinking outcomes. J Stud Alcohol 1997; 58:7–29.

10. Alcoholics Anonymous. Alcoholics Anonymous: Twelve steps and twelve traditions. New York, NY: Alcoholics Anonymous World Services, 1978.

11. Bogenschutz, MP, et al. Brief intervention for patients with problematic drug use presenting in emergency departments. JAMA Intern Med 2014; 174(11):1736–1745.

12. Patient placement criteria for the treatment of substance-related disorders, rev. 2nd ed. (ASAM PPC-2R; 12). Chevy Chase, MD: American Society of Addiction Medicine.

13. Richmond JS, Berlin JS, Fishkind AB, Holloman GHJr, Zeller SL, Wilson MP, Rifai MA, Ng AT. Verbal de-escalation of the agitated patient: Consensus statement of the American Association for Emergency Psychiatry Project BETA De-escalation Workgroup. West J Emerg Med. 2012 Feb; 13(1):17–25.

14. Peppers MP. Benzodiazepines for alcohol withdrawal in the elderly and in patients with liver disease. Pharmacotherapy. Jan-Feb 1996; 16(1):49–57.

15. Nielsen J, Graff C, Kanters JK, Toft E, Taylor D, Meyer JM. Assessing QT interval prolongation and its associated risks with antipsychotics. CNS Drugs Jun 1 2011; 25(6):473–90.

16. Carvalho M, Carmo H, Costa VM, Capela JP, Pontes H, Remião F, Carvalho F, Bastos M de L. Toxicity of amphetamines: an update. Arch Toxicol Aug 2012; 86(8):1167–231.

17. Hamilton HE, Wallace JE, Shimek ELJr, Land P, Harris SC, Christenson JG. Cocaine and benzoylecgonine excretion in humans. J Forensic Sci Oct 1977; 22(4):697–707.

18. van Amsterdam J, Brunt T, van den Brink W. The adverse health effects of synthetic cannabinoids with emphasis on psychosis-like effects. J Psychopharmacol Mar 2015; 29(3):254–263.

19. Ross EA, Reisfield GM, Watson MC, Chronister CW, Goldberger BA. Psychoactive "bath salts" intoxication with methylenedioxypyrovalerone. Am J Med Sep 2012; 125(9):854–858.

20. Burgess C, O'Donohoe A, Gill M. Agony and ecstasy: A review of MDMA effects and toxicity. Eur Psychiatry Aug 2000; 15(5):287–294.

21. Rosse RB, Collins JPJr, Fay-McCarthy M, Alim TN, Wyatt RJ, Deutsch SI. Phenomenologic comparison of the idiopathic psychosis of schizophrenia and drug-induced cocaine and phencyclidine psychoses: A retrospective study. Clin Neuropharmacol Aug 1994; 17(4):359–369.

22. Iseger TA, Bossong MG. A systematic review of the antipsychotic properties of cannabidiol in humans. Schizophr Res Mar 2015; 162(1-3):153–161.

23. Cole JC, Sumnall HR. Altered states: The clinical effects of Ecstasy. Pharmacy Ther Apr 2003; 98(1):35–58.

24. Pennings EJ, Leccese AP, Wolff FA. Effects of concurrent use of alcohol and cocaine. Addiction Jul 2002; 97(7):773–783.

25. Brown CG. The alcohol withdrawal syndrome. Ann Emerg Med May 1982; 11(5):276–280.

26. Pétursson H. The benzodiazepine withdrawal syndrome. Addiction Nov 1994; 89(11):1455–1459.

27. Tetrault J, P O'Connor P. Management of opioid intoxication and withdrawal. In The ASAM Principles of Addiction Medicine, 5th ed. Ed. R. Ries et al. Philadeplphia: Wolters Kluwer, 2014.

28. Clark A, et al. A systematic review of community opioid overdose prevention and naloxone distribution programs. J Addict Med 2014; 8(3).

29. Kerr D, et al. Randomized controlled trial comparing the effectiveness and safety of intranasal and intramuscular naloxone for the treatment of suspected heroin overdose. Addiction 2009; 104:2067–2074.

30. Chou R, et al. Methadone safety: A clinical practice guideline from the American Pain Society and College on Problems of Drug Dependence, in collaboration with the Heart Rhythm Society. J Pain 2014; 14(4):321–337.

31. Gossop M, et al. Factors associated with abstinence, lapse, or relapse to heroin use after residential treatment: protective effect of coping responses. Addiction Oct 2002; 97(10):1259.

32. Stolbach A, Hoffman R. Acute opioid intoxication in adults. Uptodate.com, 2014.

33. Mee-Lee S, Shulman G, The ASAM criteria and matching patients to treatment. In The ASAM Principles of Addiction Medicine, 5th ed. Ed. R. Ries et al. Philadeplphia: Wolters Kluwer, 2014.

34. Kolodny A, et al. The prescription opioid and heroin crisis: A public health approach to an epidemic of addiction. Annu Rev. Public Health 2015; 36: 559–574. Farrell G, et al. Alpha 2 adrenergic agonists for the management of opioid withdrawal. Cochrane Database System Rev 2014; 3:CD002024.

35. King N, et al. Determinants of increased opioid-related mortality in the United States and Canada, 1990–2013: A systematic review. Am J Public Health, Aug 2014; 104(8):e32–e42.

7

Evaluating the Geriatric Patient

DENNIS M. POPEO AND DIDIER MURILLOPARRA ∎

CASE HISTORY

Initial Presentation: A 63-year-old white man presented to the psychiatric emergency room with feelings of depression, stating: "Nobody wants me and I want to kill myself." He expressed feelings of hopelessness. He reported that he had "no energy" to engage in his usual hobbies, and even when he did, he took no pleasure in them. He reported a poor appetite and noted some weight loss, but could not tell how much. He reported that he has endured these symptoms for "many years," but recently his symptoms have become worse. He reported that he has not bathed in weeks, and does not have any clean clothing to wear. When asked if he had a plan to harm himself, he grew silent. He denied hallucinations and paranoid ideation upon questioning.

He appeared disheveled, malodorous, with a long unkempt beard, untrimmed nails and dirty clothes. He was alert and oriented, but showed impaired concentration, thought blocking, and diminished memory on mental status examination. His affect was depressed, constricted, and he expressed significant negativism.

He reported that he used to be employed as a porter, but lost his job over a year ago due to company downsizing. Since then, he has been struggling to meet the rent for his apartment and received an eviction notice a couple weeks prior to presenting to the hospital. He also mentioned being married and having a daughter but has been estranged from his family for over 10 years. For the past few weeks he has been living in the streets and reported having no friends or family whatsoever.

Clinical Pearl

Many psychosocial factors have been found to contribute to the onset of depression in older adults. Life events such as the death of a significant other, loss of employment, sudden medical illness, physical and emotional trauma, or homelessness are risk factors for the development of late onset depression. Social isolation and/or lack of emotional support can also exacerbate symptoms of existing depression.[1] For example, the prevalence of suicidal ideations and suicidal attempts among homeless individuals with mental illness is startlingly high, with those finding themselves homeless for the first time in their lives are at the highest risk.[2] When working with older adults, it is important to recognize that their individual social situation may contribute to the onset of their mood symptoms.

Past Psychiatric/Medical History: The patient denied any history of psychiatric conditions or past psychiatric hospitalizations. However, he presented to the psychiatric emergency room only a few hours after being discharged from the hospital. He had been admitted to the neurology service one week prior to presentation for evaluation of bilateral leg weakness and progressive fatigue, as well as urinary and fecal incontinence. While in their service, he was found to have multiple neurological deficits, including blindness of the left eye, unstable gait, exaggerated lower extremity reflexes, and decreased muscle strength. He was also noted to have impaired memory and cognitive function.

Medical history was also significant for hypertension, cardiovascular disease, and multiple strokes. He also reported a history of alcohol abuse, but denied drinking in the past six months due to lack of funds. He was started on antihypertensive and antilipid medication and discharged with follow-up appointments to the neurology clinic.

Laboratory tests and toxicology screens were negative for non-organic causes of neuropathy. Imaging of his brain revealed severe chronic microvascular ischemic disease, white matter changes, cerebral volume loss, ventricular enlargement, and extensive lacunar infarcts.

Clinical Pearl

It is not uncommon to see mood disorders and other psychiatric conditions in patients who suffer from chronic medical illnesses. This is especially true in elderly patients, given the greater incidence of arthritis, malignancies, and cardiovascular and neurodegenerative diseases in this patient population. Many of these medical conditions can mimic symptoms of depression (i.e., hypothyroidism), while others may serve as biological (i.e., stroke) and/or psychosocial (i.e., disability leading to impaired functioning and social isolation) risk factors for the development of depression in late life.[1,3] Vascular disease, in particular, poses a severe risk for the development of depression later in life, as evidenced by MRI studies of elderly patients with new onset of mood disorders.[3]

Similarly, elderly patients with depression are likely to present with multiple somatic complaints. Musculoskeletal pain, gait abnormalities, fatigue, behavioral changes, and a decline in memory and cognition are common findings in depressed older patients, even when they don't report feelings of sadness.[4] Patients and physicians may wrongly attribute new somatic and mood symptoms to a worsening of their physical illness, rather than to the onset of depressive syndromes. This means that elderly patients with physical illness are at a higher risk of delayed diagnosis or inadequate treatment of their depression. In the emergency psychiatry setting, it is important to first rule out reversible causes of mood symptoms, such as substance use, hypothyroidism, medication changes, and so forth. In addition, a careful assessment of the patient's current and past medical history, social history, and mental status is necessary in order to accurately identify the correct etiology of their symptoms and better determine management.

To Admit or Not to Admit?

This patient's presentation is not uncommon in the psychiatric emergency department setting. Factors such as social isolation, low socioeconomic status, homelessness, substance abuse, and chronic medical conditions place elderly patients at a higher risk for the development or exacerbation of depressive symptoms and other psychiatric conditions. Suicide attempts are also more common in the elderly than in the general population and are more likely to be successful due to a decline in overall health and social isolation, making rescue attempts less likely to be successful.[5] Similarly, depression in the elderly has been shown to potentiate the symptoms and worsen the prognosis of several medical comorbidities. This is especially true when there is apathy, lack of motivation, decreased interest in self-care, and impaired cognitive function, all of which may prevent patients from attending to their activities of daily living; that is, taking their medications or attending medical appointments.

This patient's presentation was concerning, since he appeared severely depressed and expressed passive suicidal ideations. His physical appearance demonstrated a loss of interest in self-grooming and personal hygiene, which puts into question his ability to take care of himself. The fact that he had lost both his job and his apartment point toward a decrease in functioning in the community, which could have been exacerbated by alcohol use. The patient also exhibited decline in cognitive functioning and memory, as well as difficulty walking and vision problems, which would have made it difficult for him to move around the city in search of a shelter. He had previously stated that he would not take the medication prescribed during his hospitalization or attend his follow-up appointment, stating, "What's the point?"

This patient's depression and cognitive limitations are evidently causing severe functional impairment, making him unable to take care of his basic needs. This patient is at significant danger to self and would benefit from admission while the etiology of his depression is assessed further.

Disposition: Given the patient's recent hospital stay, most of the medical workup to rule out secondary causes of depression had already been performed and were within the normal limits. The only significant medical finding was his multiple strokes and cerebrovascular changes on MRI. Neuropsychiatric testing showed that despite the patient's chronic cerebrovascular disease, his cognitive function was not severely impaired, making vascular dementia less likely. The patient was admitted to the psychiatric unit for treatment of severe depression.

DISCUSSION

Epidemiology and Clinical Features

While the prevalence of major depressive disorder (MDD) in the elderly is lower than that in younger adults (~1% vs. ~12%), many older adults experience depressive symptoms without meeting criteria for a specific depressive syndrome.[6] As the elderly population in the United states continue to grow, it is expected that the prevalence of MDD and other depressive disorders in people above the age of 65 will increase as well. Thus, these symptoms will continue to be a major cause of impaired physical, mental, and social functioning in late life.[7] Elderly patients commit approximately 20% of all suicides in the United States, with depression being the most common cause. Also, elderly patients discuss suicide less openly, they use more violent methods, and their attempts are more likely to be lethal.[6,7]

Depression in geriatric patients can be categorized into early-life-onset depression (EOD) and late-life-onset depression (LOD), differentiated primarily by their age of onset, arbitrarily set as before the age of 50 and after the age of 50, respectively.[5] While the diagnostic criteria remain similar for both EOD and LOD, elderly patients with EOD have been found to have more first-degree relatives with depression, which suggests a heavier genetic component.[5] On the other hand, LOD is more strongly associated with other comorbidities, such as generalized anxiety disorder, memory loss, cognitive impairment, psychosis, medical illness, and cerebrovascular abnormalities.[6] LOD may also have a lower response rate to treatment, a more chronic course, and a poorer prognosis, given its association with degenerative brain processes that could be linked to age-related cognitive decline and dementia.[7]

In the emergency room setting it is important to differentiate between symptoms that could be caused by depression from those caused by other medical or psychiatric conditions. For this reason it is important to understand the patient's symptoms, psychosocial history, and medical history.

- Symptoms
  - Elderly patients with depression often present complaining of fatigue, musculoskeletal pain, difficulty walking, memory problems, and other somatic complaints. Altered mental status and psychosis may also be seen in these patients, making it complicated to identify their depression as the main etiology.
- Psychosocial history
  - As already noted, elderly patients are at an increased risk of experiencing depressive symptoms due to changes in their day-to-day lives and functionality. Increased rates of chronic medical conditions, a high number of prescription medication used, increased isolation from their families, disability, substance abuse, homelessness, and death of family and friends are some of the possible mediating and moderating factors in depressed older patients.
- Medical history
  - Depressive symptoms may be caused or worsened by various acute and medical conditions. Cardiovascular disease, liver and renal damage,

electrolyte abnormalities, abnormal thyroid function, and neurological deficits can play a role in how the patient presents to the hospital. It is also important to note the effect of medication or other substance in a patient's mood.

Evidence-Based Treatment

Treatment of depression in elderly patients depends on the specific etiology. Ancillary information such as laboratory values, brain imaging, neuropsychological testing, and collateral information from family or caregivers may be needed to appropriately diagnose the patient.

Treatment for major depressive disorder (MDD) includes a combination of antidepressant medication (Selective serotonin reuptake inhibitors (SSRI) are more commonly used than tricyclics (TCA) and psychotherapy (Cognitive Behavioral Therapy, Interpersonal Therapy, Dialectic Behavioral Therapy, etc.). Patients with severe MDD or partial remission may require augmentation of this basic treatment. If the patient presents with psychotic depression, a combination of antidepressants and antipsychotics is needed, and the patient may require Electroconvulsive Therapy (ECT) if agitation or suicidality are also present.

Medical comorbidities need to be addressed, and the patient should be stable medically to make rule out the possibility of an organic cause of his symptoms. There must also be a lot of care in choosing the specific medication that can be used in these patients, since they may be more susceptible to dangerous side effects, medication interactions, and overdoses.

REFERENCES

1. Bruce, ML. Psychosocial risk factors for depressive disorders in late life. Biological Psychiatry; August 1, 2002; 52(3): 175–184; doi: 10.1016/S0006-3223(02)01410-5.
2. Desai, RA., Liu-Mares, W., Dausey, DJ. Suicidal ideation and suicidal attempts in a sample of homeless people with mental illness. The Journal of Nervous and Mental Disease; 2003; 191(6): 365–371.
3. Krishnan, KRR. Biological risk factors in late life depression. Biological Psychiatry; August 1, 2002; 52(3): 185–192; doi: 10.1016/S0006-3223(02)0349-5.
4. Gallo, JL., Rabins, PV. Depression without sadness: Alternative presentations of depression in late life. American Family Physician; September 1, 1999; 60(3): 820–826.
5. Thompson, DJ., Borson, S. Principles and Practice of Geriatric Psychiatry, 2nd ed. Chapter 25: Major depression and related disorders in late life. Philadelphia: Lippincott Williams & Wilkins. 2011, 349–365.
6. Lapid, MI., Rummans, TA. evaluation and management of geriatric depression in primary care. Mayo Clinic Proceedings; 2003;78: 1423–1429.
7. Schinka, JA., Schinka, KC., Casey, RJ. Suicidal behavior in a national sample of homeless veterans. American Journal of Public Health; 2012; 102: S147–S153; doi: 10.2105/AJPH.2011.300436.

8. Brown, RT., Kiely, DK., Bharel, M. Geriatric syndromes in older homeless adults. Journal of General Internal Medicine; August 2011; 27(1): 16–22; doi: 10.1007/S11606-011-1848-9.

9. Alexopoulos, GS., Borson, S., Cuthbert, BN. Assessment of late life depression. Biological Psychiatry; 2002; 52: 164–174.

10. Livingston Bruce, M., Seeman, TE., Merrill, SS. The impact of depressive symptomatology on physical disability: MacArthur Studies of Successful Aging. American Journal of Public Health; November 1994; 84(11): 1796–1799.

11. Sneed, JR., Culang-Reinlieb, ME. The vascular depression hypothesis: An update. American Journal of Geriatric Psychiatry; February 2011; 19(2): 99–103.

12. Brown, RT., Kiely, DK., Bharel, M. Factors associated with geriatric syndromes in older homeless adults. Journal of Health Care for the Poor and Underserved; May 2013; 24(2): doi: 10.1353/hpu.2013.0077.

8

Personality Disorders as a Psychiatric Emergency

WIKTORIA BIELSKA AND GILLIAN COPELAND ∎

A personality disorder is defined in psychiatric terms as a long-term pervasive pattern of maladaptive behaviors that have reached a degree of severity that they interfere with normal functioning. In contrast to, for example, an acute depressive episode where a patient has a discrete period of mood symptoms, patients with either a full-blown personality disorder or maladaptive personality traits have sometimes life-long patterns of thought and behavior that interfere with their ability to work and form relationships. While patients with paranoid, schizotypal, avoidant, obsessional, or schizoid traits may present to the ED for various reasons, borderline, narcissistic, and antisocial patients are by far the most frequent source of ED presentations and also cause the most distress for providers and families. It is usually not possible to diagnose someone with a personality disorder based on one brief encounter in the ED, but recognizing patterns of behavior and gathering longitudinal history can be helpful in informing disposition and treatment.

CASE 1: AFFECTIVE DYSREGULATION AND "ACTING OUT"

Case History

Ms. A is a 26-year-old single woman who is a graduate student. She was brought by an ambulance to the emergency room by a therapist at her school's student mental health service after she told the social worker she wanted to kill herself. She showed the social worker a bottle of clonazepam and asked if there were enough pills to kill herself. The meeting with the therapist had occurred because the patient's roommate brought her to the student mental health service after she told the roommate she was planning on killing herself.

The patient reported compliance with her medications of lamotrigine, escitalopram, and aripiprazole. She reports that she started feeling "bad" in the last week when her "only friend" told her he was taking a job in another state and her roommate told her she planned to move to a different apartment when the lease was up. The patient says of the experience, "Everyone is leaving me, I don't want to live anymore." She expressed surprise that she had been brought to the hospital and asked to be discharged as she was "feeling better." When asked what she thought would happen when she showed her therapist a bottle of medication and asked if it was enough to kill her, she reluctantly agreed that the therapist had done the right thing. She explained that she had immediately felt better when "my therapist saved me," and now no longer felt suicidal and wanted to leave. She denied any substance use, which was corroborated by her roommate. There was no evidence of psychosis or mania on exam. She had not engaged in any superficial self-injury in several years.

Past Psychiatric History: Ms. A has been hospitalized several times for suicide attempts including overdosing on several SSRI pills and one episode of stabbing herself. She has been on various medications and has largely been compliant with them, although has been limited in what she can take because of severe "side effects." She has never been psychotic or manic, according to information provided by her psychiatrist. She has been in dialectical behavioral therapy in the past and found it very helpful; however, her current insurance plan mandates she be treated in the student health clinic, which does not provide that service.

Past Medical History: None.

Social/Developmental History: Ms. A was eager to share that she grew up as the only child of two parents. Her father died when she was young and her mother remarried. She experienced sexual abuse by her step-father for several years as a teenager. She graduated from college and was now in graduate school. She was not married and not currently in any romantic relationships, although she could not describe the nature of the relationship between her and the "friend" who was moving to a different state.

Laboratory Studies: Urine toxicology was negative for THC, cocaine, PCP, barbiturate, benzodiazepines, opiates, and methadone. Blood alcohol level was zero. Other laboratory studies were unremarkable.

To Admit or Not to Admit?

The patient had been functioning well up until this acute stressor, which seemed to be precipitated by her intense fear of abandonment by her friend. She did not have any acute symptoms apart from this episode, but she did have a significant history of prior suicide attempts. A case could be made for either admission or discharge.

Disposition: Her outpatient treaters were not comfortable taking her back for treatment unless she was observed further and a safety plan was made. Ms. A remained unwilling to engage in any constructive planning, becoming more irritable and refusing to engage at all. She was admitted to ED observation for crisis stabilization, as the psychiatrist was concerned that an inpatient admission would be counterproductive but was also concerned about the lack of supports. Unfortunately, she became angry and hostile when told she would be staying in the hospital for the night and demanded to leave. She started throwing food at staff and other patients, threatening to throw chairs. She could not be verbally redirected but did accept sedating medication to take by mouth. She slept for the night.

The following morning she apologized for her behavior and was able to talk about her feelings of emptiness when she learned that her friend and roommate was "leaving" her. She was able to engage in a reasonable discussion about safety planning, including allowing her therapist to hold on to her clonazepam and meeting more frequently with her therapist. Her outpatient treaters were in agreement with this plan and made an appointment for her to be seen immediately upon release from the ED.

CASE 2: THE BLOODY KNIFE

Case History

Mr. P is a 37-year-old man recently divorced and employed as a massage therapist. He recently moved from the suburbs to the city following his divorce. He was brought to the hospital by ambulance after his ex-wife called 911 from outside of the city. According to EMS, the patient had texted a photograph of a bloody knife to his ex-wife and then was not answering the telephone when she called him. She was concerned and called an ambulance. On exam, Mr. P appears incredulous that he is in the emergency room and says, "all of a sudden, emergency crews showed up in my apartment and the police said they would handcuff me if I didn't come with them." He was angry about being in the emergency room, repeatedly demanding that he be allowed to leave before an evaluation could be done. After accepting an explanation about the emergency nature of his evaluation and that he would not be permitted to elope from the emergency room, Mr. P calmed down and was able to engage in an interview. He continued to insist that he had no complaints and had no idea why he was in the emergency room. When the evaluator shared with him the history provided by EMS, Mr. P admitted that he had texted such a picture to his ex-wife. He went on to explain that he had felt very upset by the divorce, even though he initiated it. He had noticed on social media earlier that day that she was tagged in a photo with a different man. He was at home cutting a beet root to roast for dinner when he noticed the way it looked like blood on his knife. He thought it looked "cool" so he took a picture and texted it to his ex-wife. When evaluator confronted him about not returning any phone calls from his ex-wife, he said he was "tired." He remained "confused," stating, "I just don't understand what all the fuss is about." He expressed anger at his ex-wife for "doing this to me." He denied suicidal or homicidal thoughts, denied symptoms of depression other than difficulty sleeping since moving into the city alone. He did admit to feeling "lonely" at times, as much of his social network was in his old town. He had been in psychotherapy before, but since moving to the city, he has not been in psychotherapy. He denied any drug or alcohol use.

Past Psychiatric History: Mr. P has never been hospitalized for psychiatric reasons. He has engaged in superficial self-injury in the past, most recently 6 months ago in the context of his divorce. He has never made a suicide attempt and stated he has never been violent or arrested. He was in psychotherapy for many years but not currently. He reports a long history of disrupted relationships where after an initial intense period of involvement, the relationship falls apart in a dramatic way.

Social History: Divorced, no children, employed as a massage therapist. Mr. P does not drink alcohol, use drugs, or smoke cigarettes currently but admits to past episodes of alcohol and cocaine use in the context of romantic relationships where his girlfriend regularly used those drugs.

Laboratory Studies: Urine toxicology negative for THC, amphetamines, benzo-diazepines, opiates, and methadone. Blood alcohol level 0.

To Admit or Not to Admit?

While it is possible that the patient does in fact harbor some suicidal thoughts or violent ideation towards his wife, and a period of divorce can be a risky time, particularly in a patient with a history of self-harm, there does not seem at this time to be any evidence apart from the texted "bloody knife" photo that the patient is experiencing any acute symptoms. It would be difficult to justify an involuntary psychiatric admission based on one photo, and the patient does not exhibit symptoms of an acute mood or psychotic disorder that would require inpatient treatment.

Disposition: Multiple attempts were made to confront Mr. P with the nature of his behavior and its connection with 911 being activated. He maintained that he did not understand "the fuss." He did admit that when he saw the picture of his ex-wife and another man, he felt "a little" suicidal for a moment, but had no intent or plan to act on that thought. He expressed pride that he had not resorted to cutting himself, as he had done in the past. He adamantly denied any suicidal ideation over the past months. When he was presented with an empathic understanding of his predicament regarding the intense feelings of anger at his ex-wife, his own loneliness in a new city, and perhaps his desire to hurt her in some way, he was able to acknowledge that his behavior was aggressive and expressed embarrassment at his behavior. After a careful consideration of his risk assessment, he was discharged with referral to a psychotherapist to help him with improved coping skills.

DISCUSSION: BORDERLINE PERSONALITY PATHOLOGY IN THE EMERGENCY DEPARTMENT SETTING

Diagnostic Criteria and Clinical Features

Borderline personality disorder (BPD) is a pervasive pattern of instability of interpersonal relationships, self-image, affects, and behavior which begins before age 18, manifests in a variety of contexts, and results in significant impairment of functioning.[1] It is a serious psychiatric illness, characterized by instability in relationships, self-image, and emotions, often leading to impulsivity and self-damaging behavior. Common and important features are a severely impaired capacity for attachment, predictably maladaptive behavior in response to separation, and a lifetime suicide rate of 10%.[2] Given the brevity of assessment and acuity of presentation, it is much more common for the ED psychiatrist to see patients who display features or traits that are consistent with borderline pathology than to be able to actually diagnose someone with the disorder. It is also important to understand that patients in the throes of an acute mood or psychotic episode may display traits or symptoms that are not consistent with their lifetime personality structure, and clinicians risk overdiagnosing personality disorders in the acute setting. However, mindfulness to personality pathology and its powerful influence on behavior remains helpful in determining treatment and outcome.

In the Emergency Department

Although there is limited data evaluating the BPD in the ED setting, given the rates just described, it is a common co-occurring condition in ED visits, particularly in patients who have repeat the ED visits.[3] Individuals with BPD are high utilizers of medical care: while studies have demonstrated a prevalence of about 1–2% of the general population, BPD has a prevalence of 6% in primary care settings, 10% of psychiatric outpatients, and 20% of inpatients.[4-6] For the ED psychiatrist, evaluating and treating the patient with BPD carries its own set of challenges, particularly around risk assessment, management of countertransference (personal as well as institutional), and determination of appropriate disposition. Key to understanding BPD in the ED setting is that individuals with BPD tend to experience the world as chaotic, and thus experience emergencies. Furthermore, there is a high co-occurrence of substance abuse, eating disorders, re-traumatization, depression, chronic suicidality, and self-harm behaviors, all of which lead to ER visits. Recurrent suicidal or self-injurious behavior is one of the diagnostic criteria, so it should be not be a surprise that there have been estimates that 43–80% percent of those diagnosed with BPD engage in some type of self-mutilating behaviors (e.g., cutting, burning, skin picking, head banging).[7] Typically such behaviors are primitive maneuvers to manage intense feelings rather than as suicide attempts.[8] Although these behaviors are often to manage intense emotional states, rather than cause death, they can be potentially lethal. Frequent self-mutilators were found to be more likely to attempt suicide, and it is important to keep in mind the high rate of completed suicide attempts (10%), either through the fatal outcomes of misadventure or through intentional suicide. Because of these factors, the crises that bring a patient with BPD into the ED are often difficult to manage, and clinical and medicolegal complications may arise.[9] However, the task of the emergency room psychiatrist remains the same: to determine whether hospitalization is required and what treatment (medication or otherwise) should be prescribed.

Management of Countertransference

As discussed in the chapter 15 of this volume, "Psychodynamic Aspects of Emergency Psychiatry," countertransference can be understood as the set of reactions and feelings that clinicians experience, whether consciously or unconsciously, in response to a patient's presentation in the context of their own history and background. Countertransference is frequently thought of as something negative, but clinicians who are aware of their own reactions and triggers can use these feelings as another assessment tool.

Patients with BPD are often difficult to manage in the emergency setting. The hallmark symptoms of BPD, such as volatile emotions, dangerous behaviors, and a tendency to escalate, are often the exact factors which make staff wary.[10] While these patients often make provocative statements that can ring false, not paying enough credence to the patient's subjective sense of crisis (whether or not it seems realistic to the listener) can have poor outcomes. It is useful to keep in mind that the maladaptive behaviors that we see were developed in response to a particular environment, and patients with BPD can be hypersensitive to perceived rejection, criticism, or negativity. Anxiety around being poorly treated is a common trigger for acting out, and patients may appear labile, needy, and easily frustrated.[11]

It is common for staff members to feel as though they are being deliberately provoked, challenged, or manipulated by these patients. In the case of Mr. P, he minimized the circumstances leading to 911 being called and was initially demanding to leave, no doubt confusing and frustrating the interviewer. His behavior could raise the concern that he is engaging in intimidating behavior toward his ex-wife, in a more classically antisocial way. Ms. A endorsed highly variable emotions within the context of the interview, making it difficult to formulate her present state of mind. While such interactions can be provocative, there are some clear guidelines that can go a long way in managing the particular needs of these patients. For example, by establishing early on that staff is invested in helping, we can lessen anxiety. Encouraging the patient to identify and explore the precipitants that lead to crisis, interpreting their impulses as a reaction to overwhelming feelings that may no longer be present, and supporting the decision to visit the PED instead of acting on destructive impulses can shift the paradigm so that the individual is enabled to control his or her impulses. Having a frank discussion about what the patients need and want from the ED visit can lessen fears of abandonment. When needed, limits should be clear, reasonable, and enforceable. Clinicians should be mindful of their tone of voice, volume, and rate of speech, as individuals with BPD are often very perceptive of negative attitudes conveyed by nonverbal communication.[12] Refraining from engaging in power struggles and choosing to "agree" on less important issues allows the focus to remain on patient safety and collaboration.

Considerations for Risk Assessment

Risk assessment in this population can be challenging, given the level of distress they often present, the seriousness of their comorbidities, and the lethality of the diagnosis. Furthermore, there is no consensus about indications for hospitalization of patients with BPD that are having a psychiatric emergency. The American Psychiatric Association 2001 Practice Guidelines indicate brief hospitalization when patients present an imminent danger to others, lose control of suicidal impulses or make a serious suicide attempt, have transient psychotic episodes, and have symptoms of sufficient severity to interfere with functioning.[2] Given the common presentation of patients with BPD, one reading of the guidelines could suggest that most presentations would lead to hospitalization. However, common practice over the years has suggested that patients with personality disorders regress on inpatient units, do not benefit from admission, and that hospitalization is counter therapeutic.[10,13,14]

A key part of the borderline experience is that affective dysregulation is often time limited. There is recent work that shows that short-term hospitalization, such as a brief crisis center admission or extended ED observation, may be the best alternative to classic psychiatric inpatient hospitalization.[15] Providing a "hold" can treat acute symptoms, which are often time limited; allow for management and mitigation of acute risk, including bridging to social supports and long-term treatment; and enable short therapeutic interventions, including validation of patients' subjective distress, attention to situational stressors, and limit setting, which introduces the issue of accountability and diminishes the potential for destructive effects on others.

However, there are specific times when hospitalization is the appropriate treatment choice. Special consideration for admission should be made in the following circumstances: complete absence of outpatient support; after potentially lethal suicide attempts; and when a comorbid mood or psychotic disorder is driving the symptomatology and is currently untreated. Furthermore, given that the risk of completed suicide increases with number of prior attempts,[16] admission should be seriously considered for an individual with a history of serious and potentially lethal suicide attempts who remains actively suicidal. In these cases, the presentation can be formulated as a failure of current treatment, and admission can provide time for a diagnosis of treatment failure and establishment of improved outpatient care.

Psychoeducation

For many years it seems to have been common practice for the diagnosis of BPD to be withheld from the patient. While this may have been initially a result of certain strictly analytic styles of treatment, it may also reflect a clinician's discomfort with their own negative feelings about the patient's behavior. In some patients where the diagnosis is clear and established, it can in fact be helpful for patients to be educated about the symptoms of the disorder and the hope for successful treatment if they are able to engage in therapy.[10] It is important to assess how patients understand their own problems and can be helpful to provide feedback about their behavior. For example, Ms. A had been in a structured treatment for BPD before, and reminding her of her prior diagnosis could be helpful for her in understanding her own behavior in a crisis situation and prompt her to use more effective coping skills in the future. Mr. P was able to comprehend that his behavior might have been a way of managing his own difficult feelings about his divorce. The idea that other people struggle with such intolerable feelings and emotions can be helpful and normalizing to patients who have spent their lives feeling that they are tortured and no one understands them. Furthermore, reiterating that there is growing evidence that effective treatment is available[11] that can lead to symptom improvement, increased functioning, and remission can provide needed hope and motivation to engage in outpatient treatment.

CASE 3: "MISS, DO YOU EVEN KNOW WHAT YOU ARE DOING?"

Case History

Mr. N is a 58-year-old, divorced, homeless, unemployed white man who presents to the emergency room having called 911 on himself because, "I'm suicidal." He is vague when describing how long he has been feeling suicidal, but eventually acknowledges to the doctor that he has been suicidal "for a really long time, Miss." He is unable to explain why he sought emergency services in this very moment. He pan-endorses all symptoms of depression, although on exam he does not appear depressed. In fact, he has bright and reactive affect. He also reports drinking alcohol almost daily, at least a pint of vodka. He does not believe that his drinking is a problem, rather, his understanding is that the problems is, "my depression, Miss." He has not sought outpatient treatment for his depression, despite several previous presentations to the ED that resulted in referrals to an outpatient clinic. He says that even though his drinking is not a "big problem," he does plan to go to rehab because, "they can find me housing." Following a gentle confrontation about the disconnect between his future-oriented statement about going to rehab and his statement that he is "suicidal," he says to the doctor, "You are too young to be doing this, do you even know what you're doing? Don't you understand that if you discharge me, I'll kill myself?" He then stormed out of the interview room. He was observed several minutes later reading the newspaper. He did not provide any phone numbers for collateral contact information. Staff overheard him talking on the phone about having been "kicked out" of his friend's apartment earlier that day.

Past Psychiatric History: Mr. N has had many visits to the emergency room, typically when he is intoxicated and reporting suicidal thoughts. He usually retracts his suicidal statements after spending the night. He has a history of two suicide attempts in the past, both while intoxicated. The first was after his separation from his wife. He was found by a friend about to jump out of a high story window and was hospitalized psychiatrically. The second was one year ago when he lost his apartment. He took an overdose serious enough to require a medical admission followed by psychiatric admission.

Mr. N drinks alcohol almost daily. He has been to rehab once and remained sober for a few weeks after discharge. He has no history of withdrawal seizures or delirium treatments. He has never disclosed, but it is suspected that he lost his housing, job, and wife due to his ongoing alcohol use.

Past Medical History: The patient has mild chronic elevation of his hepatic enzymes. He has never followed up with recommended ultrasound of his liver. He is mildly anemic.

Social/Developmental History: Mr. N grew up in an intact household where he experienced physical and emotional abuse from his mother. He readily discloses this information and freely discusses how he feels he had a terrible mother. He graduated from college and worked for some time in a high-paying job in finance. He has no children and he has been divorced from his wife for 20 years. He lost his job about 10 years ago and lived off his savings until about one year ago when he ran out of money. He lost his apartment around that time and has been intermittently staying with friends and going to shelters. He has no contact with his ex-wife or any of his family members.

Laboratory Studies: Blood alcohol level was not obtained until several hours after arrival, when it was zero. The patient refused to submit urine for a toxicology screen.

To Admit or Not to Admit?

Although he was not grossly intoxicated when he came in and although his remarks about suicide were not consistent with the exam (i.e., he had bright affect and was future-oriented despite reporting depression and suicidal ideations), there is more than meets the eye with Mr. N. He likely did feign or exaggerate his symptoms in order to have a place to spend the night, and his repetitive use of the ED, ostensibly as a place to stay, could also seem antisocial in nature. However, a decision about his disposition and treatment is an exercise in countertransference management. The decision needs to be based on a strict consideration of his risk factors for danger-ousness rather than the desire to be as far from him as possible, a sensation he likely induces in most people, as evidenced by his limited social supports. Ignoring the feelings of hatred he engenders, we see that he has multiple serious risk factors for suicide, including his age, gender, race, substance use, history of significant suicide attempts, and poor social supports. His suicide attempts in the past have occurred in the context of significant stressors like losing his primary relationship and his housing. Added to these static risk factors are his current intoxication (albeit mild) and the recent stressor of being kicked out of his friend's home. He is at relatively high risk for suicide. While most of his risk factors are not changeable, his intoxica-tion is changeable by being observed longer. It is also important to note that con-fronting the patient during the interview may have acutely injured him, in that he perceived that the clinician doubted him and therefore possibly thought negatively of him, which is intolerable to him. A need to "prove" to the clinician how serious he is may then acutely worsen his risk of self-harm.

Disposition: Mr. N was placed on hold overnight to monitor for withdrawal and to monitor his behavior for any evidence of depressed mood. The following morning he retracted his suicidal statements and asked to be discharged. He said he planned to go to a different friend's apartment in the morning. He was encouraged to go to detox and rehab, both of which he declined. He was offered a referral to outpatient substance abuse treatment but said he was not planning on going. He showed no signs of alcohol withdrawal at time of discharge.

CASE 4: THE "MISUNDERSTANDING"

Case History

History of Present Illness: Ms. D is a 34-year-old, married, employed, black woman who works as a freelance designer and has no past psychiatric history. She was brought by an ambulance after her fiancé called 911 when he walked in on her putting her head in the oven. He also discovered that she had purchased a firearm recently and was worried she would use it to kill herself. She actually has a husband (who she married for immigration purposes and does not have a relationship with now), a fiancée (with whom she has been "engaged" for the last five years; he financially supports her and she lives in his apartment, but they no longer in a romantic relationship), and a boyfriend (with whom she has a roman-tic relationship). She is indignant about being brought to the emergency room and explains that her fiancé has entirely "misunderstood" the situation. She ex-plains that he has recently asked her to move out of his apartment and told her he would no longer be supporting her financially because he would like another woman to move into his apartment. She says, "Yeah, I'm not happy about the situation, but I'm happy for him for moving on. I've just been stressed out about where I will move to. Wouldn't you feel this way?" She denied any symptoms of depression, including sleep and appetite disturbance, low mood, or suicidal thoughts. She adamantly denied she had made or was thinking of making a suicide attempt.

She is very resistant to anyone speaking to her fiancé, the person who activated EMS. She refuses to provide his collateral contact information, but he calls the emergency room himself to speak with the doctor. He explains that when he told her she would need to move out one month ago she laughed at him and said she would rather die than have to live in a less expensive part of town. Since then she has been increasingly withdrawn and irritable with him. He believes she has made a résumé to apply for jobs but has not been submitting résumés, fearing she will be rejected. What has concerned him recently is her secretiveness. He discovered her on the day of presentation with her head in the oven after he returned home from work a few hours earlier than usual—she was not expecting him to be home at that time. He is also puzzled about her recent purchase of a firearm as she has never expressed interest in owning or using a gun. He is extremely concerned about her safety. He has not observed any symptoms of depression apart from her irritability.

Past Psychiatric History: Ms. D has never seen a psychiatrist before and has never been psychiatrically hospitalized. She has seen a therapist in the past to help her with "relationship troubles." She has no history of suicide attempts.

Ms. D does not drink alcohol or use drugs. This was corroborated by her fiancé.

Past Medical History: None.

Social/Developmental History: Ms. D refused to talk about her early developmental history ("that's none of your business") but did say she has no children and explained the relationship situation described previously. She graduated from college and initially worked at several large prestigious firms where she was "let go" after working a few months because, "they didn't value me." She currently works for herself with moderate success attracting clients to her design services.

Laboratory Studies: Blood alcohol level was zero. Toxicology screen was negative.

Mental Status Exam: Ms. D is an attractive, pleasant, agreeable, young woman dressed in stylish clothes and makeup. She is polite and deferential to the physician, if somewhat overly familiar. She frequently asks for validation that that physician would share her feelings if presented a similar situation. She is linear and logical in her thought process, adamantly denies that she is suicidal, and minimizes the circumstances that prompted EMS activation. She repeatedly says, "You have to get me out of here, doctor, I'm not like these other patients."

To Admit or Not to Admit

Ms. D's presentation is very concerning. She has taken steps to conceal her suicide attempt from her fiancé/roommate and had no reason to expect him home early. Furthermore, she has recently purchased a firearm, suggesting a plan to kill herself. It is notable that other than some social withdrawal, there are no symptoms of depression described either by the patient or the person she lives with. This is an important finding in a narcissistic patient. Often the suicidal thoughts are related to feeling rejected not because of struggles around abandonment as in a borderline patient, but because the rejection is a confirmation of a fear of worthlessness. In this case, there is also a potential of a loss in social status (moving to a less prestigious neighborhood, having to rely only on her more meager income). Although she lacks major historical risk factors for self-harm, such as history of self-harm and drug use, her recent stressor and recent efforts to conceal her suicide attempts make her at moderate to high-risk for suicide.

Disposition: Ms. D was admitted to the hospital on an involuntary basis. She was enraged at the admission and difficult to treat throughout her stay.

NARCISSISM AND NARCISSISTIC PERSONALITY DISORDER IN THE EMERGENCY DEPARTMENT

When most people think of someone with narcissistic personality disorder (NPD), they think of an arrogant, haughty person. This stereotype misses not only the true clinical picture of NPD, which can be quite diverse, but also the significant suffering people with NPD can experience. As the vignettes demonstrate, NPD presents significant diagnostic and management challenges in the emergency setting.

NPD describes a pervasive and debilitating pattern of interpersonal relationships, self-image, and affects marked by grandiosity, need for admiration, and lack of empathy. Narcissistic personality disorder affects anywhere from 1 to 6.2% of the population.[17] It is associated with significant comorbidities, including substance abuse and depression.

The difficulty in understanding the pathology is that unlike the apparent uniformity of the diagnosis as presented in DSM-V, there are several different subtypes.[18,19,20] The criteria captured by DSM-V capture important aspects of the pathology but may not be helpful in capturing all or even most individuals who receive the diagnosis in clinical practice. The subtypes that seem to emerge are the grandiose, "overt," subtype; the vulnerable, "covert," subtype; and the healthier, "higher functioning" subtype.[19] Although the complexities of diagnosis may be outside the scope of an emergency setting, it is important to consider NPD or narcissistic traits in not just patients that seem "narcissistic" in the colloquial sense. For instance, Ms. D was likeable, polite, and not obviously grandiose. She struggled with feeling "unvalued." The physician's experience of her was not entirely negative, although her interpersonally exploitative relationships might have roused feelings of anger.

Diagnosis of any personality disorder, including NPD, can be very difficult. There are no quick and reliable instruments.[21] Furthermore, the emergency setting allows only for assessment in one point in time, while a diagnosis of personality disorder requires understanding a patient more longitudinally. The diagnostic criteria are specific that this must be a "pervasive pattern" that has been present since late adolescence/early adulthood. Crises and emergency situations lend themselves to bringing out pathological traits in a person who may be able to function at a higher level when not in crisis. While understanding the narcissistic character is important in understanding a patient in the emergency room, it is important not to assume the patient is always organized narcissistically unless there is a known pattern or history.

A narcissistic patient is particularly sensitive to appearing vulnerable or powerless, a common feeling among patients in the emergency department. When her fragile sense of self is threatened in this manner she can become provocative and devaluing, thereby jeopardizing the opportunity for complete assessment. As illustrated in the case of Ms. D, the personality pathology can complicate a thorough assessment in many ways. Ms. D may have both consciously and unconsciously distorted the history to make herself appear in the best light. Collateral information was crucial in this case, in finding information that made an accurate risk assessment possible. In the case of Mr. N, he may feel such humiliation about his homelessness and social situation that just saying he feels distressed about his circumstances may feel impossible. The vulnerability may feel intolerable to him. Instead, he engages in manipulative and provocative statements designed to get a night in the emergency room, a behavior consistent with the interpersonally exploitative style of NPD patients.

Managing Countertransference and Building Rapport

The interpersonal difficulties that NPD patients suffer from can generate difficult feelings (or countertransferences) in nurses, staff, and physicians in an emergency department. Feelings that clinicians may struggle with in the emergency setting when treating NPD patients include feeling used, feeling bored, and feelings of hatred, among many others. Some literature has described clinicians left feeling unreasonably idealized, devalued, or disregarded.[17,19] Often, the feelings evoked are intense and difficult, reflecting both the severity of the patient's pathology and the intensity of the patient's emotional experience in a time of crisis. Awareness of these feelings is the first step in managing a difficult encounter and ensuring the best possible assessment. Processing difficult feelings about a patient encounter with colleagues can alleviate their intensity and help provide the necessary perspective to provide the best patient care.[21]

Building a good therapeutic alliance can go a long way to help stabilize the patient and assess his functioning. Clear, respectful gestures enable the patient to maintain his positive sense of self. Whereas other patients might benefit from a more familiar tone, the NPD patient will often respond best with respectful formalities such as "sir" and "thank you for speaking with me."

Much can be accomplished in terms of building rapport with an NPD patient by accepting and tolerating the patient's negative affect (often manifesting as difficult behavior) without reacting in a retaliatory way.[22] For instance, Mr. N's devaluing statements toward the clinician including, "You are too young to be doing this," and "Do you even know what you're doing?" could create a temptation to act in a defensive or retaliatory manner. In remaining neutral and respectful, the clinician can avoid a power struggle and complete the evaluation.

In addition, setting clear expectations for behavior and firm but respectful limit setting can also make the patient feel better and help him avoid sabotaging the evaluation. The limit setting is easier for the patient to accept when paired with identification and validation of his feelings. For instance, if Mr. N's devaluing had continued, the clinician could have said, "It can be frustrating not to know someone's credentials when your health is at stake, but if you can't speak to me respectfully I will have to terminate the interview."

Treatment

The treatment of personality disorders, including NPD, is not done in the emergency room or even in the hospital. Treatment requires long-term psychotherapy.[18,22,23] Despite this, patients with personality disorders are frequent utilizers of emergency psychiatric services. There is limited research into the prevalence of personality pathology in emergency room contexts, but a Swiss study found that patients with a personality disorder were four times more likely than patients with mood, anxiety, substance use, or psychotic disorders to have recurrent visits to the psychiatric emergency room during the study period.[24] The reason for patients with personality disorders in particular using the emergency room more frequently are yet to be fully understood. It is likely that the often limited family and social supports, as well as comorbidities including mood disorders and substance use, lend themselves to frequent crises. Complicating the possibility of engaging in appropriate outpatient treatment are the interpersonal difficulties of personality disordered patients. For NPD patients in particular, engaging in an outpatient treatment that requires a commitment, respecting the boundaries of the therapist, and accepting set appointments can be difficult.[18,25]

Whether or not narcissistic problems alone bring patients to an emergency room, narcissistic pathology is worth diagnosing and considering, as NPD patients are also likely to seek emergency treatment related to comorbid diagnoses. The narcissistic pathology could make the assessment and treatment of other co-occurring diagnoses challenging.

It is thought that because NPD is associated with ego-syntonic symptoms such as feelings of superiority rather than suicidality and self-injury, narcissistic individuals are less likely to seek treatment. Newer literature suggests that NPD patients, particularly more vulnerable subtypes, can be help seeking. Many of these patients are distressed and lonely with poor social functioning.[26]

Differential Diagnosis and Risk Assessment

In addition to evaluating comorbid disorders, identifying and properly evaluating NPD patients in the emergency room is important for risk assessment. Having a personality disorder increases risk for suicide, particularly a Cluster B personality disorder.[27] For NPD patients in particular, the risk for suicide could be from poorly managed comorbid conditions (i.e., mood disorders, substance use) or part of the personality pathology itself. For instance, NPD patients may find that their focus on beauty, fame, and wealth have been disappointed when they reach midlife or older age. This could precipitate a crisis.[20,28] NPD, in particular, seems to pose a risk for suicide after being fired from a job, supporting the idea that diminished fame or perceived importance may lead to crisis.[29] Furthermore, suicide attempts in attempters diagnosed with NPD are characterized by higher lethality and are less impulsive.[30]

A study that followed patients with personality disorders for 10 years found that of all the personality disorders that seemed to confer risk of one suicide attempt, only NPD predicted a number of suicide attempts beyond the initial attempt.[31]

Just as with any personality disorder, NPD patients can have comorbid mood and psychotic disorders. Importantly, suicide risk does not seem to necessarily correspond with the presence of or severity of mood symptoms.[30] As discussed previously, managing co-morbid illness can also be hindered by the presence of NPD, making it difficult to manage some of the modifiable risk factors.

In summary, although NPD and narcissistic traits are associated with ego-syntonic symptoms such as feelings of superiority rather than suicidality, the reality of NPD is a more complex clinical picture of often very vulnerable patients who are at risk for suicide. Often these patients make a careful evaluation and risk assessment challenging because of the difficult feelings they create in physicians, nurses, and staff. Maintaining a neutral and respectful attitude, obtaining collateral information, and carefully thinking through risk assessment are important aspects of emergency evaluation of NPD patients. Unlike a borderline patient, who wants the clinician to see how distressed he feels, a narcissistic patient may conceal difficult, embarrassing, or painful feelings. She is also more likely to have a lethal suicide attempt without obvious symptoms of depression.

Key Clinical Points

- Evaluating patients with prominent personality pathology can be complicated and engender uncomfortable feelings in the clinician and lead to incomplete assessments or acting out, i.e., deviating from an accepted framework of assessment or disposition.
- Acutely dysregulated patients may be able to be stabilized with a brief "hold" or observation that avoids regression in the inpatient setting.
- Personality disorders are debilitating. BPD carries a greatly increased risk of self-harm and completed suicide.
- Narcissistic patients may make suicide attempts in the absence of a mood or psychotic syndrome in response to what they perceive to be intolerable threats to their self-esteem.

REFERENCES

1. American Psychiatric Association, DSM Task Force. Diagnostic and statistical manual of mental disorders: DSM-5. 2013; http://dsm.psychiatryonline.org/book.aspx?bookid=556.
2. American Psychiatric Association. Practice guideline for the treatment of patients with borderline personality disorder. *American Journal of Psychiatry.* Oct 2001; 158(10 Suppl):1–52.
3. Ellison JM, Blum NR, Barsky AJ. Frequent repeaters in a psychiatric emergency service. *Hospital & Community Psychiatry.* Sep 1989; 40(9):958–960.
4. Torgersen S, Kringlen E, Cramer V. The prevalence of personality disorders in a community sample. *Archives of General Psychiatry.* Jun 2001; 58(6):590–596.
5. Gross R, Olfson M, Gameroff M, et al. Borderline personality disorder in primary care. *Archives of Internal Medicine.* Jan 14 2002; 162(1):53–60.

6. Leichsenring F, Leibing E, Kruse J, New AS, Leweke F. Borderline personality disorder. *Lancet (London, England).* Jan 1 2011; 377(9759):74–84.

7. Stanley B, Brodsky B. Risk factors and treatment of suicidality in borderline personality disorder. *Clinical Neuroscience Research.* 2001; 1(5):351–361.

8. Dulit RA, Fyer MR, Leon AC, Brodsky BS, Frances AJ. Clinical correlates of self-mutilation in borderline personality disorder. *The American Journal of Psychiatry.* Sep 1994; 151(9):1305–1311.

9. Pascual JC, Corcoles D, Castano J, et al. Hospitalization and pharmacotherapy for borderline personality disorder in a psychiatric emergency service. *Psychiatric Services (Washington, D.C.).* Sep 2007; 58(9):1199–1204.

10. Perlmutter RA. The borderline patient in the emergency department: An approach to evaluation and management. *The Psychiatric Quarterly.* Fall 1982; 54(3):190–197.

11. Oldham JM. Guideline watch: Practice guideline for the treatment of patients with borderline personality disorder. 2005, Arlington, VA.

12. Gilbert SB. Psychiatric crash cart: Treatment strategies for the emergency department. *Advanced Emergency Nursing Journal.* Oct-Dec 2009; 31(4):298–308.

13. Beresin E, Gordon C. Emergency ward management of the borderline patient. *General Hospital Psychiatry.* Sep 1981; 3(3):237–244.

14. Paris J. Is hospitalization useful for suicidal patients with borderline personality disorder? *Journal of Personality Disorders.* Jun 2004; 18(3):240–247.

15. Berrino A, Ohlendorf P, Duriaux S, Burnand Y, Lorillard S, Andreoli A. Crisis intervention at the general hospital: An appropriate treatment choice for acutely suicidal borderline patients. *Psychiatry Research.* Apr 30, 2011; 186(2-3):287–292.

16. Ansell EB, Wright AG, Markowitz JC, et al. Personality disorder risk factors for suicide attempts over 10 years of follow-up. *Personality Disorders.* Apr 2015; 6(2):161–167.

17. Stinson FS, Dawson DA, Goldstein RB, et al. Prevalence correlates, disability, and comorbidity of DSM-IV narcissistic personality disorder: Results from the wave 2 national epidemiologic survey on alcohol and related conditions. *J Clinical Psychiatry.* 2008; 69(7):1033–1045.

18. Ronningstam EF. Narcissistic personality disorder: A Clinical perspective. *Journal of Psychiatric Practice.* 2011; 17:89–99.

19. Caligor E, Levy KN, Yeomans FE. Narcissistic personality disorder: Diagnostic and clinical challenges. *American Journal of Psychiatry.* 2015; 172(5):415–422.

20. PDM Task Force. Psychodynamic diagnostic manual. Silver Spring, MD: Alliance of Psychoanalytic Organizations, 2006.

21. Tyrer P, Reed GM, Crawford MJ. Classification, assessment, prevalence, and effect of personality disorder. *Lancet.* 2015; 385:717–726.

22. Yeomans FE, Levy KN, Caligor E. Transference focused psychotherapy. *Psychotherapy.* 2013; 50(3):449–453.

23. Ronningstam EF. Narcissistic personality disorder. In: Gabbard, GO, ed. Treatments of psychiatric disorders. 5th ed. Arlington, VA: American Psychiatric Association; 2014:1073–1086.

24. Richard-Lepouriel H, Weber K, Baertschi M, DiGiorgio S, Sarasin F, Canuto A. Predictors of recurrent use of psychiatric emergency services. *Psychiatric Services.* 2015; 66:521–526.

25. Hengartner MP. The detrimental impact of maladaptive personality on public mental health: A challenge for psychiatric practice. *Frontiers in Psychiatry.* 2015; 6(87):1–10.

26. Miller JD, Campbell WK, and Pilkonis P. Narcissistic personality disorder: Relations with distress and functional impairment. *Comprehensive Psychiatry*. 2007; 48:170–177.

27. McGirr A, Alda M, Seguin M, Cabot S, Lesage A, Turecki G. Familial aggregation of suicide explained by Cluster B traits: A three-group family study of suicide controlling for major depressive disorder. *American Journal of Psychiatry*. 2009; 166:1124–1134.

28. Jahn, DR, Poindexter, EK, Cukrowicz, KC. Personality disorder traits, risk factors, and suicide ideation among older adults. *International Psychogeriatrics*. 2015; 1–10.

29. Blasco-Fontecilla H, Baca-Garcia E, Duberstein P, et al. An exploratory study of the relationship between diverse life events and specific personality disorders in a sample of suicide attempters. *Journal of Personality Disorders*. 2010; 24(6):773–784.

30. Blasco-Fontecilla H, Baca-Garcia E, Dervic K, et al. Specific features of suicidal behavior in patients with narcissistic personality disorder. *Journal of Clinical Psychiatry*. 2009; 70(11):1583–1587.

31. Ansell EB, Wright AG, Markowitz JC, et al. Personality disorder risk factors for suicide attempts over 10 years of follow-up. *Personality Disorders: Theory Research, and Treatment*. 2015; 6(2):161–167.

9

Evaluating and Treating Children with Psychiatric Complaints in the Emergency Department

RUTH S. GERSON AND FADI HADDAD ■

CASE 1: "I CAN'T HANDLE HER ANYMORE"

Case History

Erica is a 15-year-old girl who is brought to the emergency room by her foster mother. Erica's foster mother reports that she cannot handle Erica anymore due to her oppositional attitude, refusal to follow rules or go to school. She also notes overall odd behavior especially when the foster father is around. Erica has lived with this foster family for the past 3 months, and the foster mother knows very little about Erica's life before that. Before coming to live with them, Erica was described as calm, polite and pleasant, but within 2 weeks the family saw changes in Erica's behavior. She seemed disinterested in spending time with the family, even for fun activities, and became very oppositional and even hostile when the foster parents asked her to do something, even basic things like going to school. When the foster father was home, Erica isolated herself in her room and did not interact much with him; a few times when the foster mother went to check on her, she saw Erica talking to herself. The foster agency was informed and they tried to refer Erica and the family to therapy but the foster parents were not able to attend due to their work schedule, and Erica never talked much with the therapist.

On arrival to the ED, Erica seems entirely disinterested, answering questions mostly with a shrug or a one-word answer. She says that she does not like the foster family nor her school and that she would rather go to a different family and be home schooled. She denies being depressed or sad, but when asked questions about her past, she becomes tense, then tearful. When asked about psychotic symptoms, she states that she hears voices telling her that she is a loser and bad, and sometimes other voices telling her to run away from home. She denied any thought of harming herself or others.

Past psychiatric history: Neither the family nor Erica were able to inform us about Erica's past. But we contacted the foster agency who told us that Erica was born to a single mother who was a drug addict, and father was unknown. Child protection removed Erica from home after she was found in a car alone, crying and screaming, at the age of 2 months, while her mother was buying drugs on a street corner. Erica has lived in 8 foster homes. In each one, she had a honeymoon period where she seemed like a perfect child and then started acting out. At age 9 Erica disclosed that her prior foster father had raped her and threatened her if she disclosed it; she was terrified and did not tell anybody until 2 years later. She was sent for therapy but she did not engage with the therapist. She started cutting school and acting up at home, and has had five more foster placements since then.

Medical History: Erica's delivery was normal, though not is much known about her pre-natal care or in-utero drug exposure. She was a healthy baby, and per the foster care records she met her developmental milestones 1–2 months later than expected but with no serious difficulties or delays.

Social Development: Erica has some friends at school, but she had lots of fights with them. She was described as being either provocative, instigating fights and conflicts with peers, or totally the opposite: isolated, aloof and not interested in any of the other students. Academically she was doing well until last year. The school social worker observed Erica to be more isolative last year; when the social worker investigated she realized that Erica was being teased and sexually harassed by an older male student. The student was removed to a different class so Erica did not have to interact with him.

Family History: Not much is known about the biological family. In the current foster family, the mother is a stay-home mother, and the father a fireman, with two younger biological children. The parents are affectionate but strict with their children in regards to their behaviors and school achievements.

Laboratory Studies: General labs, including CBC, electrolytes, liver function, and thyroid function tests, were normal. Urinalysis, urine pregnancy, and urine screen toxicology were negative.

Clinical Pearl

Erica's case shows how complicated diagnosis for adolescents can be in the emergency room. On the surface, Erica presents with behavioral problems (oppositionality, breaking rules, cutting school) and possible psychosis (isolating, talking to herself, hearing voices). This could be suggestive of conduct disorder or a psychotic disorder, but with a better understanding of her social situation and history, we see a much more complex presentation. She was born to a neglectful, drug-addicted mother and may have been exposed in-utero to drugs or other stressors. She was removed from her neglectful mother at a very early age but then had multiple foster care placements since then, disrupting any opportunity for her to develop attachment to a care giver. She has been sexually abused by a foster parent, then bullied at school, and has had minimal positive relationships with either peers or adults. When her symptoms are considered in light of these risk factors, she may be experiencing posttraumatic stress disorder (PTSD) with avoidant (social isolation, school refusal, avoiding contact with foster family) and reactive (oppositionality, fighting at school) reactions to trauma reminders. She could also be experiencing a severe depression, and the voices that she reports could be part of a mood disorder, a symptom of PTSD, or a way that she has learned to describe her own negative thoughts and urges.[1]

To Admit or Not to Admit?

Disposition: This patient is denying suicidal thoughts and has not shown any dangerousness to others, but on the other hand her presentation is very complex and she is not functioning in the community. She does not feel safe neither at home nor at school and has severe enough symptoms which requires intensive treatment to target her PTSD symptoms, investigate further any depressive symptoms and understand the etiology of the "voices" that she hears to ensure she is not truly psychotic. If the patient felt safe at home and felt connected to an outpatient therapist, treatment outside of the hospital could be feasible, but in this case she should be stabilized in the hospital and then connected to intensive outpatient treatment.

CASE 2: "DANGER TO SELF AND OTHERS"

Case History

John is a 16-year-old boy who is brought to the emergency room by ambulance from school for "danger to self and others." John was in history class when the teacher gave him an assignment to read aloud to the class; John did not want to do this, started arguing with the teacher, and then began yelling and screaming and throwing his books on the floor. The referral letter from the school indicated that John has been deteriorating in his functioning at school and has been hanging out "with the wrong crowd."

Upon arrival to the ED, John was calm, cooperative, and open in discussing the event that brought him to the ED. He stated that most of the time, he is unable to focus in the classroom. He daydreams and does not understand the instructions for his homework. He tries to entertain himself but always gets in "trouble" with others. He also finds reading particularly difficult. He says he did not want to read the assignment in class because he had been daydreaming and did not know where in the text he was supposed to start, and also because he feels embarrassed when reading in front of others. He has been having problems with focus and reading for the past two years but lately he feels that it is affecting his work much more than before. In the past 6 months, he has been hanging out with older group of peers. He admitted that he has been trying cigarettes, MJ, and some other substances they offered him. He claimed that he is calmer when he smokes. He denied any changes in his mood, sleep, or appetite.

Past Psychiatric History: John had no other psychiatric problems and no past treatment, but his mother notes that he's always had some difficulty with school work, and that she had to help him much more than his siblings to get his homework done. She says his work takes him much longer than she thinks it should and that he seems to get distracted very easily.

Medical History: John was born in a normal delivery after a normal pregnancy. Developmental milestones were normal. He had no major medical problems or any history of head trauma.

Social Development: John manages with others but he does not have many friends. He gets easily frustrated when he has to wait for his turn and gets into fights and arguments with others.

School History: John has historically been an average student, but it seems that he is finding school more difficult every year. He was always easily distracted but was able to keep up with his homework with the help of his mother. On his report cards, his teachers would often say that John was smart but not focused or not applying himself.

Family History: No psychiatric family history is reported, but John's mother stated that his father had similar issues at school when he was John's age.

Laboratory Studies: Labs were normal, except that the urine toxicology was positive for THC.

Clinical Pearl

John has multiple symptoms of untreated ADHD—his distractibility, daydreaming, inability to follow instructions, difficulty waiting turns, social immaturity, and impulsivity.[2] He also may have a learning disability in reading. John's presentation from school is very common for adolescents with untreated ADHD and learning disabilities.[3] His difficulties have gone unnoticed because he is a fairly bright child whose mother has been giving him a lot of extra help, but as the academic requirements of school increase with each year, he has been struggling more and getting more and more frustrated. John's untreated ADHD is also a risk factor for substance abuse, both because he is more prone to impulsive decisions (such as accepting drugs when offered) and because with his problems at school and with his peers, he has found that using drugs is one of the few ways he can fit in and feel accepted.

To Admit or Not to Admit?

In this case, while the school was concerned about "danger to self and others" because of his agitation at school, by the time John arrived to ED he was calm and cooperative, with no evidence of any suicidal or homicidal thoughts, so he does not need inpatient admission. But if John's untreated ADHD and academic needs are not addressed, he is likely to have a similar outburst at school very soon. John should be referred to an outpatient clinic in order to have a full evaluation for ADHD. There he should be evaluated both for medication and also for school accommodations to help him succeed academically.[3] Social issues and interactions should be addressed through individual therapy or through social skills group therapy. A thorough evaluation should be done for the substance abuse to determine the amount he is using and to provide the appropriate treatment.

CASE 3: HITTING THE TEACHER

Case History

Todd, a 7-year-old boy, is brought by ambulance to the ED from school after becoming extremely agitated, screaming, and hitting teachers. Todd had been playing with a toy airplane he had brought in for show-and-tell, and when asked to put the toy away and pay attention to the class, Todd refused. When the teacher attempted to take his toy, Todd became very agitated and combative, and even with the teacher and two safety officers, he could not calm down. Todd is in a special education classroom for ADHD but just joined this classroom two weeks ago after his parents and teachers agreed on a change to his Individualized Education Plan (IEP).

His current teacher and the one from his old classroom agree that since he came to this school a year ago, Todd has always been quite odd. He does not have friends and does not interact much with others, except to tell them about his favorite topic: airplanes. He seems not to care if the other person is interested in airplanes or not and gets very upset when asked to change the topic or to participate in any other activity. Most of the day, he spends the time by himself, reading his own books, but refusing to do his assignments. Over the two weeks since changing classrooms, he has been in the principal's office every day due to agitation.

Todd's mother stated that he had language delays. He received early intervention services, including speech therapy, because he did not speak until age three, and then received ongoing speech and occupational therapy until age five. He improved and after that he enrolled in a regular education kindergarten, but he has always had behavior problems and never seemed to make friends. His mother worried something was wrong, but the pediatrician never gave any diagnosis other than the ADHD.

Past Psychiatric History: No other history than indicated above.

Medical History: No medical problems.

Social Development and School History: As above.

Family History: No family psychiatric history.

Laboratory Studies: No laboratory abnormalities.

Clinical Pearl

It is unusual for a young child to be brought to the ED for dangerous behavior, so when that happens, it is often a red flag that something big is going wrong in the child's life (such as abuse, a big disruption at home such as parents' divorce or a parent's death, or a psychiatric disorder that has gone untreated).[4] In Todd's case, he meets criteria for an untreated autism spectrum disorder: he had speech delays at an early age, has always had social communication difficulties, has a restricted interest in airplanes, and is rigid in his thinking and response to challenges or changes in routines (such as a change in the classroom).[2]

To Admit or Not to Admit?

A child like Todd needs specialized treatment, but an inpatient hospitalization is unlikely to be helpful, as the sudden change in routine and separation from family is likely to be very stressful for him and thus worsen his behavior further.[5] Todd should be referred to a treatment center for autistic youth that can provide intensive, specialized outpatient treatment including applied behavioral analysis therapy (ABA), social skills groups, and an educational evaluation for placement in a specialized school for children with autism.

DISCUSSION

Child psychiatric emergencies are, by their very nature, deeply complex.[5,6,7] Psychiatric crisis in a child almost always involves family members, schools, peer dynamics, and the complexity of the child's cognitive, social, and emotional development. Even defining an "emergency" in children can be more complicated. There may not be immediate danger to self or others, but rather, a situation where the adults in the child's life cannot keep him or her safe (or are actively harming the child, as in cases of child abuse or neglect) or where the child or family is lost in the system without treatment or guidance. The variety of cases we see in the emergency room shows that even knowledgeable and dedicated parents, teachers, and therapists can find themselves at a loss, at times, with these complex cases.

The fact that children cannot always express the triggers for their behavior or the reasons for their distress due to their cognitive, emotional, and developmental abilities makes the process of the evaluation even more difficult. The most obvious "guess" of an explanation for a child's behavior is rarely the right one, and involving parents, teachers, school staff, and other providers to fully understand the stressors in the child's life is crucial in making the assessment. The information from all parties might not match. The complexities of the different aspects of the child's life that can cause the child to act differently at home, school, or in any other setting depends on the child's sense of safety, and of being heard and cared for, in those environments, as well as the different demands of those different settings. For example, if a child feels that his teachers care about him and that he is managing socially with peers he might present with no problems at school while his life at home could be described as a nightmare due to witnessing violent conflicts between parents or living in extreme poverty. A child with an undiagnosed learning disability could suffer at school from frustration, embarrassment, and teasing from peers, while at home he lives with a loving, caring parent who tries her best to provide for him; he too will show very different symptoms and behaviors at home compared to school. If the school sends him to the emergency room for an outburst and the only collateral obtained is from his mother and not from school staff, this will not be a complete assessment.

Gathering the information from every provider and setting is not easy, particularly in the limited time available for an emergency evaluation. Often the child's therapist, teachers, or guidance counselors will not be available at the time of the evaluation, and we will have to make a decision to hospitalize or discharge the child home based on the incomplete information at hand. To make the best assessment with these limitations, the emergency child psychiatrist must use all of her observational skills to fill in the gaps in the story. Ideally, the staff should observe the child from the moment he enters the emergency room. For example, a child who sits next to his mother in the waiting room while the mother is trying to soothe him, feed him, or talk to him probably feels safe and heard by his parent and thus is likely to calm down more quickly than a boy who sits away from his mother, refusing any eye contact or comfort. Observing the parent or teacher that accompanies the child also tells much about the child's supports and resources. Is the adult trying to distract or soothe the child, or are they busy texting or complaining to other parents while their child seethes. Observing the way the child separates from the parent to come to the interview also speaks to anxiety and sense of security.

The next critical step of the assessment is to attempt to take the child's perspective to identify the triggers for the symptoms and behaviors to determine how they can be modified.[1,3] An aggressive outburst in a child such as Todd, in the third case, is motivated by rigidity, obsessional interests, and sensory overstimulation, not by a desire to injure someone or by paranoid ideation.[8] Such triggers are rarely immediately obvious, and the child is often unable to describe them. With detailed description from teachers and parents of the events leading up to the outburst and of the child's behaviors and functioning overall, the clinician can put together a hypothesis of what might be going on. When such a hypothesis is floated to the child with a tone of curiosity and empathy, the child will feel respected and understood and will often calm down quickly. The clinician can then help the parent, teacher, or other adult to understand the child's perspective so that the family, school, and child can problem solve together.

Often the greatest challenge to managing child psychiatric emergencies is not the child, but helping the family and school to come to terms with the challenges the child is facing and find the help the child needs. Families presenting to the ED with a child in psychiatric distress are often in crisis, which either contributes to the child's distress or is triggered by it. Helping the parents or caregivers to understand what is going on and manage their own emotions (which often range from anxiety to guilt to frustration to fear) is the first step to helping them understand how to access the right help for their child. For a child such as Erica, in the first case, this step is particularly critical. If Erica's foster parents, agency worker, and teachers can see how her behaviors may be rooted in posttraumatic stress disorder and depression, rather than just oppositionality, they will be vastly more able to help her in future moments of crisis, and they will better understand what kind of professional help she needs.[3]

The final key piece in working with children in psychiatric crisis is assessing what treatment or professional help the patient has in the community.[1,7,9] The child's outpatient therapist, psychiatrist, or guidance counselor can provide information that is crucial to the diagnostic evaluation and safety assessment of the child. When a child does not have any treatment in the community at the time he or she presents to the ER, the emergency psychiatrist should consider the child at higher risk, as finding and connecting with community providers that treat children can take weeks or months.[10] The emergency psychiatrist or social worker can be of immense help to a child or family if they can help the family understand what kind of treatment the child needs and how to access it. The needed help may not only be psychiatric; for a child like John or Todd, in the second and third cases, the need is significant educational help and resources as well as treatment by a psychiatrist and therapist (with expertise in autism for Todd and in substance abuse for John). If this is not set up, these boys are likely to be right back in the ED.

Key Clinical Points

- Assessing children and adolescents in the emergency room requires collection of collateral information from family, school, and outpatient clinicians, as this provides crucial information for safety planning and diagnosis.
- Understanding the child's perspective with an approach that is curious and empathic is key to identifying the triggers for the crisis and how environmental factors exacerbate or uncover psychiatric symptoms.
- Families of a child in psychiatric crisis are often in crisis themselves, and they need help understanding their child's symptoms, managing their own emotions, and recognizing the child's perspective.
- Accessing effective community treatment is not easy, and children in crisis often need educational accommodations and social services as well. Emergency providers can be immensely helpful to patients if they can help families navigate the complex medical and educational services landscape (and this will also keep kids from coming right back to the ER with the same problem).

REFERENCES

1. Haddad F, Gerson R., eds. *Helping kids in crisis: Managing psychiatric emergencies in children and adolescents.* Arlington, VA: American Psychiatric Publishing, 2014.
2. American Psychiatric Association. *Diagnostic and statistical manual of mental disorders* (5th ed.). Washington, DC: Author, 2013.
3. Rappaport N, Minahan J. *The behavior code: A practical guide to understanding and teaching the most challenging students.* Cambridge, MA: Harvard Educational Press, 2012.
4. Prager N, Donovan AL. *Suicide by security blanket, and other stories from the child psychiatry emergency service.* Santa Barbara, CA: Praeger Publishing, 2012.
5. Chun TH, Katz ER, Duffy SJ, Gerson RS. Challenges of Managing Pediatric Mental Health Crises in the Emergency Department. *Child and Adol Psych Clinics of N America.* 2015; 24:21–40.
6. American Academy of Pediatrics, Committee on Pediatric Emergency Medicine; American College of Emergency Physicians and Pediatric Emergency Medicine Committee, Dolan MA, Mace SE. Pediatric mental health emergencies in the e-mergency medical services system. *Pediatrics.* 2006; 118(4):1764–1767.
7. Dolan MA, Fein JA, Committee on Pediatric Emergency Medicine. Pediatric and adolescent mental health emergencies in the emergency medical services system. *Pediatrics.* 2011; 127(5):e1356–1366.
8. King BH, DeLacy N, Siegel M. Psychiatric assessment of severe presentations in autism spectrum disorders and intellectual disability. *Child and Adol Psych Clinics of N America.* 2014; 23: 1–14.
9. Nock MK, Green JG, Hwang I, McLaughlin KA, Sampson NA, Zaslavsky AM, Kessler RC. Prevalence, correlates, and treatment of lifetime suicidal behavior

among adolescents: Results from the National Comorbidity Survey Replication Adolescent Supplement. *JAMA Psychiatry.* 2013; 70(3):300–310.

10. Olfson M, Marcus SC, Bridge JA. Emergency department recognition of mental disorders and short-term outcome of deliberate self-harm. *Am J Psychiatry.* 2013; 170(12):1442–1450.

10

Developmental Disability and Autism Spectrum Disorders in Adults

KATHERINE MALOY ■

CASE 1

Case History

Mr. S is a 35-year-old man who has lived in residential facilities for developmentally disabled individuals since the age of 10, when his family became unable to manage him at home. The patient is brought from his residence by staff and EMS personnel after he became agitated and struck at staff members. They note that usually he can be calmed by playing music or allowing him to pace, but this time he continued to follow staff and try to hit them. He also destroyed a TV set. This is very uncharacteristic behavior for the patient, who has been stable for many years.

On interview, the patient is a very tall, obese man who makes no eye contact. He is entirely nonverbal, which staff states is his baseline. He is noted to be rocking in a chair. He does not appear distressed or agitated.

Past Psychiatric and Medical History: According to paperwork accompanying the patient from the facility, he is diagnosed as having severe intellectual disability. He is also diagnosed with autism spectrum disorder. He has a history of seizures, and is maintained on a regimen of valproic acid and topiramate.

No laboratory studies were obtained, as the patient was resisting staff who approached him for blood draw and EKG.

Observation and Disposition: The patient sat calmly for a few hours with staff present and showed no evidence of agitation, although he did occasionally get up to pace and at one point was witnessed jumping up to touch the ceiling tiles. Staff at the residence note that he has had some changes in his routine at his day program and may have been more constipated lately. The director of his residence states they are unwilling to have him return tonight, and think that he should be hospitalized "because he is obviously dangerous."

CASE 2

Case History

Mr. A is a 44-year-old man who lives at home with his mother. He was diagnosed with autism spectrum disorder in elementary school and receives disability income. He is brought to the ED by his cousin for worsening self-injurious behavior and threatening statements toward the family. They note that although the patient is verbal and functions independently in terms of his activities of daily living, he is entirely dependent on his family for money management and housing. Since graduating high school with a special education diploma, he has consistently refused to attend any kind of vocational or social programming and spends his days in his room, searching the internet for images of race cars. He has a care coordinator through a local community agency who visits monthly to check on him and the family. His mother is having medical problems and has been out of the home for appointments and brief hospitalizations; his care has been taken over by the cousin and other family members. This evening the patient began slapping himself and screaming and could not be calmed down.

On interview the patient is calm, makes no eye contact and speaks in a very low and monotonous manner. He answers every question in a concrete manner, and it takes some time to elicit information from him. He eventually states that he has been having intrusive and distressing images in his mind of his mother being dismembered or decapitated and he finds these images very frightening. During the interview, while discussing this distressing content, he begins rocking, stands up, and turns in a small circle, repeating the same phrases over and over. His cousin— who has had limited interaction with the patient until his mother became ill—is very frightened by the patient's behavior, and doesn't think he can manage him at home. He admits to yelling at the patient and trying to grab his hands when he begins slapping himself, which seems to worsen the behavior.

Past Medical and Psychiatric History: Aside from evaluations when he was in school to determine his diagnosis and enroll him in benefits, he has had no contact with psychiatrists, no hospitalizations, no suicide attempts, and no history of violence. The cousin is aware of the patient having some episodes of hitting himself when angry. He has no medical illnesses but is very reluctant to attend his yearly primary care appointment.

DISCUSSION

People with intellectual disability comprise approximately 1% of the population,[1] and the prevalence of autism spectrum disorders was estimated in 2010 to be 7.6 per 1000 persons. Patients with intellectual disability or autism spectrum disorder are a particular challenge for the emergency psychiatric setting for a multitude of reasons. In patients who are nonverbal, or who have static cognitive deficits, it is difficult to assess the etiology of their distress, as they cannot report what they are feeling or thinking. Even milder deficits can lead to impaired frustration tolerance due to a decreased ability to understand social cues or interpersonal issues, as well as difficulty modulating emotions and behavior. A hallmark of autism spectrum disorder is difficulty with social interactions, but there is also great difficulty toler-ating changes, frequent obsessional or repetitive behaviors, and even if a patient is verbal, there can be difficulty expressing emotions verbally. Many patients with autism spectrum disorder have comorbid intellectual disability, many do not, but even with a normal or near-normal IQ, there can be profound deficits in social functioning. It is a mistaken perception that patients with autism do not have feel-ings, and it is easy to think that patients with severe intellectual disability do not feel or experience emotions if they are nonverbal. All of the usual tools of a psychiatrist—reading affect, relating to patients verbally, and using an interview to obtain information—can seem useless in the face of these challenges. The emer-gency or inpatient psychiatric setting itself is ovestimulating, confusing, and unfa-miliar, and patients may be vulnerable to assault or exploitation by other patients.

On a systems level, the care of patients with intellectual and developmental dis-abilities has typically been separated from the care of patients with mental illness. It is very common for states to have separate departments of "Mental Health" and "Developmental Disability." Services available for the developmentally disabled community can be difficult to access and require the patient to be diagnosed and enrolled prior to age of maturity, which in turn requires that a parent or school were attuned to the issue and it was recognized and diagnosed. Patients whose parents are undocumented immigrants and fear governmental intervention, or who choose to not send their children to school, may not be recognized as needing services until the parents become too old to care for them. Appropriate supported housing is difficult to find and frequently of low quality. Although overall there has been a strong push away from institutionalization of individuals with developmental disabilities, the community options can be limited or community residences may be unwilling or unable to manage someone who has periods of aggression or self-injury. Families can become exhausted, parents age, and circumstances change over time. Significant health care disparities exist for patients with intellectual disability, which are aggravated by systems issues, difficulty with communication, and lack of provider experience or comfort working with this population.[3] Thus, patients end up in the emergency department, and psychiatry is called to intervene.

Autism spectrum disorders also are extremely heterogeneous in their presen-tation and level of disability, which further complicates the lumping of these dis-orders with other developmental disabilities. A person with an IQ of 30 who is nonverbal, has frequent seizures, and exhibits stereotypic repetitive behaviors may be diagnosed with both intellectual disability and an autism spectrum disorder but has very different needs and issues than someone with normal IQ who attends col-lege classes but has difficulty making friends due to their obsessional need to talk constantly about airplanes.

In patients with behavioral dysregulation who are nonverbal or who are severely disabled, it is not uncommon to see psychiatric diagnoses attached to the patient that are of questionable validity. While it is certainly possible for someone with intellectual disability to have a comorbid depression, bipolar disorder, or psychosis, these labels are unfortunately used at times to justify use of psychiatric medications to treat troubling behaviors. The treatment of self-harming or aggressive behavior that is due to a static cognitive deficit, or due primarily to autism, should first be addressed through behavioral measures, such as providing a calming environment, distracting activities, addressing any physical discomfort, and having a regular, therapeutic, or educational routine. Medications may be employed as a last resort, but patients can be very sensitive to side effects, and it is difficult to comprehend how to adjust and titrate to effect with someone who cannot tell you how they are feeling.

Risperidone has been approved for the treatment of disruptive behaviors in patients with autism spectrum disorders[4] but does not address difficulties with social interaction,[5] and risks of movement and metabolic disorders should be weighed carefully. Many different pharmacotherapeutic strategies have been attempted to manage difficult behaviors or target core autism symptoms, including SSRIs,[6,] naltrexone,[7] and anticonvulsants,[8] all with varying results. Most research has been conducted in children. Patients whose behaviors are worsened due to uncontrolled seizure activity may benefit most from stabilization of their seizures, and EEG monitoring may be indicated if seizure activity is suspected in episodic behavioral disturbance.[9]

In the emergency department setting, any strategy that allows the patient to have reduced stimulation and be around familiar people or objects can be helpful in avoiding agitation or use of medications. Patients should remain with a familiar caregiver whenever possible, have access to items or activities that soothe them, and should be permitted to engage in stereotypic behaviors if they seem helpful. Staff may require some education about the nature of the patient's difficulty to help adjust the environment accordingly. Frequently patients in professional residential settings will have a written behavioral plan; with patients from home, family members can provide helpful information about the patient's preferences.

If, as a very last resort, acute pharmacologic intervention is indicated to manage behavioral that is acutely dangerous, there is little research available. Using lower doses of medications, avoiding benzodiazepines due to risk of disinhibition, and using agents with lower risk of dystonia and extrapyramidal effects are all reasonable strategies. One should also be cautious of lowering seizure threshold in patients with epilepsy or worsening co-occurring musculoskeletal issues in patients with comorbid cerebral palsy.

Disposition

In the first case, it seemed most likely that the patient's acute distress was related to changes in his environment and/or physical discomfort. There was no evidence of continuous periods of psychomotor agitation, changes in sleep, or hypersexual behavior that might indicate a mood disorder. He had a few discreet periods of uncharacteristic agitation, which were not sustained. While it is understandable that his residence is concerned about his behavior, it is also likely that time spent in an acute psychiatric setting that is unfamiliar, loud, and full of aggressive patients is most likely to worsen the patient's behavior by making him afraid and uncomfortable. The patient's residence was reminded that the patient has rights as a tenant and cannot be refused appropriate housing if hospitalization is not indicated, and they were advised to treat his constipation and try to work with his day program to reestablish his regular routine. He was also given an earlier appointment with his neurologist, and his valproate level was checked and found to be in the therapeutic range.

In the second case, the patient was observed overnight and the cousin was provided with psychoeducation about the patient's diagnosis and behaviors. The patient expressed some relief at being able to verbalize what he was feeling and while never mentioning his mother or her illness, he was responsive to reassurance that she was expected to recover from her most recent illness and would be returning home soon. He had no further episodes of slapping himself and reported that his intrusive thoughts had lessened. His care coordinator was brought in for a meeting with the team and the cousin to discuss in-home support options to allow the patient to remain in the home and to begin the process of planning for how the patient would be cared for if his mother became more ill or died. The patient was given a follow-up appointment with a psychologist from the agency that manages his care, and the care coordinator planned to increase the frequency of his visits to monitor the safety of the situation at home.

Key Clinical Points

- Although patients with autism spectrum disorders and intellectual disability have frequently been grouped together in terms of provisions for treatment and services, they are a heterogenous population and individual patients may have very different needs and ability to function.
- Behavioral interventions and modification of the environment are always the first-line of treatment when patients have disruptive or difficult behaviors.
- Evaluation of patients with limited verbal or social ability can be complicated, and collateral information about the patient's baseline and longitudinal course should be considered.
- Mood and psychotic disorders can be comorbid with intellectual disability and autism spectrum disorders, but clinicians should be careful to avoid labeling patients who do not truly meet criteria for a mental illness.
- Medical illness, physical discomfort, or change in routine can all cause behavioral changes in non-verbal patients and should be ruled out.

REFERENCES

1. Maulik P, Mascarenhas M, Mathers C et al. Prevalence of intellectual disability: A meta-analysis of population-based studies. Research in Developmental Disabilities 2011; 32(2):419–436.
2. Baxter AJ, Brugha TS, Erskine HE et al. The epidemiology and global burden of autism spectrum disorders. Psychological Medicine 2015; 45 (3):601–613.
3. Krahn G, Hammond L, Turner A. A cascade of disparities: Health and health care access for people with intellectual disabilities. Mental Retardation and Developmental Disabilities Research Reviews 2006; 12:70–82.
4. McDougle CJ, Holmes JP, Carlson DC, Pelton GH, Cohen DJ, Price LH. A double-blind, placebo-controlled study of risperidone in adults with autistic disorder and other pervasive developmental disorders. Arch Gen Psychiatry 1998; 55(7):633–641. doi:10.1001/archpsyc.55.7.633.

5. Shea S, Turgay A, Carroll A et al. Risperidone in the treatment of disruptive behavioral symptoms in children with autistic and other pervasive developmental disorders. Pediatrics Nov 1, 2004; 114(5):e634–e641.
6. Kolevzon A, Mathewson KA, Hollander E. Selective serotonin reuptake inhibitors in autism: a review of efficacy and tolerability. The Journal of Clinical Psychiatry. 2006; 67(3):407–414.
7. Roy A, Roy M, Deb S et al. Are opioid antagonists effective in attenuating the core symptoms of autism spectrum conditions in children: a systematic review. Journal of Intellectual Disability Research, Special Issue: Mental Health and Intellectual Disability. 2015; 59(4):293–306.
8. Hirota T, Veenstra-Vanderweele J, Hollander E et al. Antiepileptic Medications in Autism Spectrum Disorder: A Systematic Review and Meta-Analysis. Journal of Autism and Developmental Disorders. 2014; 44(4):948–957.
9. Myers S, Johnson C. Management of Children with Autism Spectrum Disorders. Pediatrics 2007; 120:1162–1182.

11

Ethical Issues
in Emergency Psychiatry

AMIT RAJPARIA ■

CASE 1: THE STRESSED OUT MOTHER

Case History

Tonya, a 43-year-old female arrives via ambulance to the emergency room appearing grossly intoxicated and slurring her speech. The ambulance crew report that she was picked up outside of her apartment building at 1 P.M., where she was crying loudly and stumbling back and forth. At triage, she tells the nurse to "leave me alone, just let me die." She endorses having "some vodka" that day but denies other substances. She denies doing anything to hurt herself prior to presentation. She reports a history of GERD and asthma for which she takes omeprazole and citalopram. She promptly falls asleep and, though able to be aroused, cannot readily answer questions.

Vital signs are BP 95/55, HR 52, T 98.4, R 12. She is triaged to the medical ED where she has screening laboratories drawn and continuous monitoring of her vital signs.

Clinical Pearl

When there is concern about suicidal behavior and the historian is not reliable, one should consider obtaining toxicology assays to screen for common and potentially lethal overdose agents. Although laboratories will differ, these include acetaminophen and salicylates; levels for any medications the patient may be taking or have available including lithium, valproate, carbamazepine, phenytoin, phenobarbital, or tricyclic antidepressants; in addition to testing for common substances of abuse.[1] There is additional concern in this case due to Tonya's somnolence and depressed heart rate/blood pressure, although the alcohol alone could explain these findings.

Three hours later she awakens briefly. Vital signs at that time are: BP 110/70, HR 65, T 98.5, R 14. Screening lab results are essentially within normal limits. The ED physician orders a psychiatric consultation to "evaluate suicidal ideation."

In reviewing the medical record, the psychiatrist notes two previous ED visits: one after a fall down stairs and another for abdominal pain. She also notices that on Tonya's last visit one year ago she reported having a 12-year-old daughter. Upon questioning Tonya about her daughter, she becomes frantic, asking "What time is it? I've got to get out of here. She's coming home from school soon." The psychiatrist was able to confirm that the daughter had found her way to her aunt's house after returning to an empty apartment, and reassures the patient.

Clinical Pearl

It is critical at triage to ask patients about children or elderly dependents in the home, and to assure that those dependents are safe. If Tonya's child was younger or less resourceful, the outcome could have been more troubling. If patients do have dependents, their safety should be confirmed early in the process by speaking directly with the person who is currently taking responsibility for them.

On further interview, Tonya is still slurring her speech, has a labile affect ranging from tearful to angry, and is demanding to leave. She ultimately drifts back into sleep. The psychiatrist informs the ED physician that an adequate safety assessment is not possible in her current state. He asks that the patient be continued on a 1:1 watch and that she should be held until an adequate assessment can be completed.

Clinical Pearl

When placing a patient on an emergency hold in an unlocked medical ED setting, the psychiatric consultant should be sure to consider the environment and provide recommendations for the ED staff to mitigate potential risks. For the risk of self-injury, violence, or elopement, one should consider a 1:1 watch, placing patients further away from exits, prenotifying hospital security, and providing recommendations for emergency medications in case of agitation.

The psychiatrist subsequently receives telephone calls from several family members, pleading with her to admit Tonya psychiatrically. They are afraid on a weekly basis that she is going to end up dead due to her alcohol binges and behavior when intoxicated. Moreover they are tremendously worried about her daughter. They say that Tonya is very depressed and that her depression is driving her "death wish." Just 2 years prior she was employed as an administrative assistant. She lost that job and may soon lose her apartment; she doesn't seem to care about anything anymore. When asked about specific suicidal behaviors, they do not list any in the recent past. The patient's brother tells the psychiatrist, "If you let her go, her death is going to be your fault."

On reassessment early the next morning, Tonya is calmer, more linear, and is demanding to leave. She complains about all the questions that are being asked of her and makes multiple snide remarks berating the psychiatrist but ultimately complies. She acknowledges being "a little down" for the past several months and having a lot of stresses, but says she is taking care of all of her and her daughter's needs. She says she drinks occasionally to cope with her stress but says she never drinks in front of her daughter.

To Admit or Not to Admit?

Disposition: The psychiatrist has a lengthy discussion with Tonya about what is likely an ongoing depressive syndrome that may be fueling her increased alcohol consumption. She offers the patient the option of an inpatient admission on a conditional voluntary basis, explaining all of the different treatment modalities that would be made available to her for both the depression and the alcohol use disorder. While the patient voices appreciation for the effort to help her, she says that she cannot remain in the hospital because she has to take care of her daughter, and she needs to work on finding on a job. The psychiatrist deliberates about admitting the patient involuntarily, but ultimately decides she does not meet legal criteria at that time.

The patient is provided referral information for a full range of treatment services and told she can return to the hospital at any time if she would like help getting connected with those services. Prior to her leaving, the psychiatrist consults with the ED social worker and they decide that they must file a report with Child Protective Services due to their concerns about neglect of the 12-year-old daughter in the context of repeated episodes of alcohol intoxication. When the patient is informed, she coldly says, "I will never step foot in this hospital again. I hope you know you're ruining my life—I thought doctors were here to help."

DISCUSSION

Mandatory Reporting of Suspected Abuse

All states have some form of mandatory reporting requirements for suspected abuse of children, while many states also have reporting requirements for other vulnerable populations including the elderly, intellectually and physically disabled. All mental health clinicians are mandated reporters, and can face professional consequences if they fail to report when indicated. Information that raises concern about abuse/neglect can come directly from the patient (dependent or caretaker), from witnessing physical signs of abuse, or from collateral sources. Clinicians should know how to readily access the necessary procedures and timeframes for reporting in their area. Given the complexity of the decisions and the associated emotional valence, it can be very helpful to seek consultation from a colleague about reporting decisions. Clinicians can anonymously consult with the child protective agency about the details of a case when it is not clear if a report is indicated. Hospitals also likely have risk management, legal counsel who can provide input, or may have designated social workers that have expertise in reporting decisions. It is important to document the rationale for reporting along with any consultation utilized. Clinicians are generally protected from malpractice actions based on mandated reports if they are made in good faith.

Such reporting decisions pit the ethical obligation to maintain confidentiality against that of protecting the welfare of dependents.[2] Confidentiality is foundational to the patient-clinician relationship, so it is unsettling for clinicians to expose information provided in that protected context, particularly when it can have law enforcement and custodial ramifications. However, it is clear as outlined in both legal statutes and professional organizations' ethics codes that society's value to protect dependents from abuse outweighs patient confidentiality,[3] and this obligation is codified in the mandatory reporting requirements.

For clinicians seeing patients in outpatient settings, it is standard practice to provide informed consent about mandatory reporting requirements early in the treatment relationship. In emergency settings, efforts can be made to provide informed consent about the possibility of involuntary hospitalization, the need to contact collateral sources, and mandatory reporting requirements. However, it can be more difficult in the ED given the need to manage the more urgent clinical situation or patients' inability to have this conversation due to an impaired mental status. If the concern for abuse or neglect of a dependent surfaces in the emergency department, it can be advantageous for the ED provider to make the report, thereby preserving the therapeutic alliance with the outpatient provider. The report should only include the minimal necessary clinical information needed for the state agency to accept and act on the report.

One further question is whether a patient should be informed when a report is being made. While in most places reporting can be completed anonymously, one should consider informing the patient when a report is made. These conversations can certainly be challenging. As illustrated in Tonya's case, the act of informing a patient about a report can disrupt a treatment alliance and may even result in the patient not accepting the recommended treatment. However, in other cases, the reporting can be understood as an attempt to help a parent get the necessary services for themselves and their children. In the conversation, the clinician can acknowledge the stresses and burdens stacked against the patient, and that they and other clinicians will continue to work with them to overcome these difficulties.[4] Certain circumstances compel a clinician not to inform the patient about a report. If there is a concern about the patient becoming violent when told, one might delay informing or get appropriate security back-up prior to informing the patient. Concern about imminent danger to the dependent as a result of the report is another reason to delay informing or not inform a patient about a report.

Emergency Holds, Voluntary and Involuntary Hospitalization

When the consulting psychiatrist was first called about Tonya, she was faced with a patient who was still intoxicated and had made a passive suicidal statement at triage. Tonya's impaired mental status made a thorough evaluation impossible at that point, but she was still demanding to leave. This is a common scenario in which to institute an emergency hold. Emergency holds involve the patient being retained in the ED or Psychiatric Emergency Services (PES) beyond the initial assessment, allowing for further observation, data collection, and a more comprehensive evaluation. Certain jurisdictions also have provisions for 24–72 hour extended observation beds within the PES for which many of the same principles apply. By the maximum time period for an emergency hold (which varies by state), a clinician must decide to either discharge the patient or provide the legal basis for an inpatient admission.

Emergency holds need to be supported by some concern for dangerousness if the patient were released prior to further evaluation. One should consider how the patient arrived to the ED. Patients who arrive by ambulance or with police generally raise a higher level of concern for safety, and thus warrant a longer period of observation. Dangerous behavior prior to ED presentation along with an abnormal mental status exam are other critical factors in justifying an emergency hold. Documentation should demonstrate the rationale for detaining a patient against their will.

The ethical considerations for such a hold are similar to those for any involuntary commitment (see later discussion). The use of emergency holds over inpatient admission supports the principle of employing the least restrictive alternative. Patient autonomy is bolstered by the possibility of an efficient discharge and avoiding a locked door setting. For Tonya, the emergency hold primarily allowed time for metabolism of the alcohol to the point where she could participate in a more comprehensive assessment. Other common scenarios that argue for an emergency hold or extended observation bed over a direct admission include: treating withdrawal symptoms, allowing for contact with a critical collateral source, rapid stabilization of a chronically suicidal patient after a non-serious attempt, and attempts at engagement and further data collection for a patient who is suspected of symptom exaggeration for secondary gain.

Prolonged ED stays due to lack of access to inpatient beds or specialized staff availability in the ED (as opposed to clinically based emergency holds) lead to lower quality of care and a longer overall length of stay. Given the dramatic shortage of inpatient psychiatric beds in many regions, boarding of psychiatric patients in EDs is unfortunately a common occurrence. Every effort should be made by hospital administrators and public officials to correct these systemic barriers to quality care.

Although Tonya's ED psychiatrist knew hospitalization would be a tough sell for her, she still presented Tonya with the recommended treatment plan that included a conditional voluntary hospitalization. The recommendation was made on the basis of the worsening depressive syndrome, alcohol use disorder, risky behavior, and low likelihood of initiating treatment outside of the hospital. The conditional voluntary status allows the hospital to retain a patient for a designated period of time after they express a desire to be discharged to allow for (a) adequate disposition planning, (b) reengaging the patient in further voluntary inpatient treatment, or (c) evaluation for conversion to involuntary status. The conditional voluntary is much more common than the simple voluntary status in which patients can leave at any time they wish.[5]

An important precursor for any voluntary hospitalization is to insure that the patient has adequate decision-making capacity to provide informed consent for the voluntary admission. The capacity threshold to assent to a voluntary admission is relatively low due to the low risk profile of hospitalization (compared to, for example, a complex surgical procedure.) Still, the patient should not be coerced into a voluntary admission because they lack criteria for an involuntary admission.

They should be able to voice at least a rudimentary understanding of what is being treated by hospitalization and agree to the basic elements of the treatment plan. While the voluntary admission supports the principle of employing a less restrictive alternative, admitting patients voluntarily when they are unable to give informed consent or are not in the least aligned with the treatment plan is often clinically counterproductive.

Once Tonya declined the voluntary admission, the psychiatrist was forced to contend with the decision to involuntarily hospitalize the patient. Involuntary hospitalization classically invokes the ethical principles of autonomy (individual patient self-determination) versus beneficence and nonmaleficence (maximizing the benefit and minimizing harm for the patient and society). The legal underpinnings for state civil commitment laws reflect this tension of balancing protection of individual rights with providing care for the mentally ill and protecting society at large.[6] The general evolution of civil commitment law in the United States has been toward the use of dangerousness criteria for involuntary psychiatric hospitalization, as opposed to broader "health and safety" criteria in Europe and elsewhere.[7]

The ultimate determination of the psychiatrist that Tonya did not exhibit imminent dangerousness sufficient for involuntary hospitalization is understandable. The decision was made more complicated by other factors that are often present in these assessments. One factor is the practice of defensive medicine, in which liability concerns play an overwhelming role in decision making. This practice is accentuated in the emergency setting where risk is high, time is short, and involuntary hospitalizations can be frequent. In this context, clinicians can often err on the side of hospitalization, the so-called "preventive detention" that is motivated primarily by self-protective motives on part of the psychiatrist.[8,9] No doubt Tonya's brother's threat to sue the psychiatrist lingered in her head as she contemplated allowing the patient to leave, particularly knowing that Tonya's constellation of chronic social stressors, mood symptoms, recent behaviors, and alcohol use could certainly lead to a bad outcome. Liability concerns can play out in the other direction as well when a patient's threats to bring legal action can dissuade a psychiatrist from hospitalizing them.

Another factor to consider is the role of countertransference in involuntary hospitalization decisions. Hearing that the patient had a 12-year-old daughter who was left to fend for herself due to her mother's drinking could certainly evoke strong negative feelings towards the patient. This is probably exacerbated by her condescending attitude toward the psychiatrist. Negative countertransference reactions can influence involuntary hospitalization decisions in both directions. In this case, the psychiatrist could have unconsciously stretched the limits of the law in hospitalizing the patient as a way to help the daughter or as a punitive measure against Tonya. Alternatively, patients who evoke strong negative feelings can be prematurely discharged when they still need treatment. Both the liability threat and countertransference reactions require a psychiatrist to examine their own motives and reactions as they inform an involuntary hospitalization decision. These are also situations in which it is particularly helpful to consult with a colleague or request a second opinion, and they are prime examples of why a team approach can be so useful in the psychiatric emergency setting.

CASE 2: THE FACEBOOK THREAT

Case History

Mark is a 35-year-old single white male employed as a computer programmer with no formal psychiatric history who is brought to the PES by ambulance. According to the paramedic, Mark's friend had called 911 stating that he had already been worried about him lately and then he saw that Mark had posted the statement "SOS. . . . I can't go on any more like this, I think this is the end for both of us" on his Facebook page.

On initial evaluation, Mark presents as irritable, stating repeatedly that this is a "big misunderstanding" and that "I never was really going to do anything to hurt Jennifer or myself." On further exploration, he says that he has been under a lot of stress because his ex-girlfriend Jennifer broke up with him and moved out 2 months ago. The prior night she had stopped by to pick up some items and rejected his efforts to try to speak with her. He acknowledges that this rejection enraged him, that he subsequently had several drinks at his home, and that he did fantasize about killing Jennifer. He says he wrote the Facebook posting in that moment of great anger, and perhaps as a way to get her attention. He answered in the negative to all of the questions on the standardized suicide screening tool administered at triage. He now vehemently denies thoughts to hurt anyone else, including Jennifer. He denies owning a gun or any other weapon or making any plans to obtain one.

Mark states that over the last month he has felt lonely, hopeless, has had several angry outbursts at work, and has been sleeping very poorly. He reported his alcohol use as a "beer or two after work," along with "a little bit of cocaine" and stated the previous night was an exception. He denies any formal psychiatric treatment. He remembers one previous episode of depression lasting 2–3 months in the context of a relationship break-up when he had very similar symptoms. He also recalls other times when he can have a lot of energy, be very productive at work, and not sleep as much, though he has difficulty recalling whether he was using cocaine during these times. He denies a history of suicide attempts, including aborted or interrupted attempts. He denies a history of violence or incarceration. His mother has a history of depression and his father has a history of alcohol abuse.

Initial labs are only significant for an EtOH (ethyl alcohol) level of 40 mg/dl and urine toxicology positive for cocaine.

Vital signs are BP 125/85, HR 80, R 12, T 98.4.

To Admit or Not to Admit?

Disposition: Mark was informed that a critical part of the evaluation would involve speaking with collateral contacts. He was adamant that he did not want any friends or family to be contacted, stating, "If they know about me being brought here, it is only going to make my stress ten times worse." He was told that since the ambulance report listed the name and address of the referring friend, an internet search would be utilized to locate a telephone number and speak with him, given the concerns about the patient's safety. The internet search yielded the friend's contact information, and the clinician was ultimately able to speak with both Mark's friend and his mother. While the friend was mostly helpful in confirming the exact nature of the Facebook posting, Mark's mother confirmed his reported history (with the exception that he was certainly minimizing his substance use), that he had not engaged in any suicidal or self-injurious behavior, that he does have a social network with whom he has been in contact through the recent turmoil. She also confirmed that she was not aware that Mark has any history of violence, including in the context of the relationship with Jennifer or previous girlfriends. Further, Mark was agreeable with the plan that his mother would spend at least the next 4 days with him at his apartment.

Mark was given a crisis bridging appointment for 2 days after discharge for the purposes of follow-up safety assessment, further evaluation and treatment of possible bipolar disorder, and bridging to mental health and substance abuse treatment. He was informed that if he missed the appointment and was not accessible by phone, the mobile crisis team would make an outreach visit to his apartment. Based on the assessment, the clinician decided that no further action was required to warn/protect Jennifer or contact law enforcement concerning Mark's threats of violence.

DISCUSSION

Breach of Patient Confidentiality

Protecting patient confidentiality is central to the doctor-patient relationship. Patient's concerns about privacy are often heightened in the PES because of their own sense of stigma about mental illness and the highly personal information that is being shared. The Health Insurance and Portability and Accountability Act (HIPAA) is the federal regulatory framework for protecting patient privacy. It limits a clinician's use of patient health information to the direct purpose of treatment. Exceptions to HIPAA are allowed when a clinician deems that the patient poses a serious and imminent threat to self or others.[10]

Ethically, clinicians are often faced with the difficult choice of preserving patient confidentiality versus fulfilling their duty to protect the patient and others from harm. This again reflects the conflict between the principles of autonomy and beneficence/non-maleficence. Risk assessment is a key component in clarifying this choice in the PES. In a situation when the risk for dangerousness is assessed to be low, a clinician may decide that a breach of confidentiality is not justified. The circumstances of Mark being brought in by ambulance, having made potential suicidal and homicidal statements, along with the risk factors of the relationship stressor, social isolation, and ongoing substance use places him at a higher risk for violence. Further, as is usually the case in the PES, the clinician does not have an established relationship of trust with the patient. In the PES critical pieces of the patient's report need to be verified whenever possible. On the basis of the imminent safety concern, the clinician justified breaching confidentiality and making the telephone calls to Mark's friend and mother without his consent.

While breaching confidentiality was justified in Mark's case, it was important for the clinician to remain empathic about the Mark's valid concerns about his privacy. This awareness can have a large impact on a clinician's ultimate goal of engaging the patient in an appropriate treatment plan. The patient should know he is not being singled out. Patients should know that involving collateral sources are a regular component of a PES assessment. It can even help to demonstrate for the patient a typical approach to such a call as a way of allaying their fears. For example in this case, "He is doing physically fine. I cannot discuss further details due to patient confidentiality, but I just need to ask you a few questions to ensure his safety. . . ."

It may be possible, in certain circumstances, to offer the patient some choice about which person they would like contacted. Although unpleasant when a patient continues to refuse consent, it is preferable to disclose the need and justification for contacting collaterals prior to making the calls, unless one deems that the patient could become violent as a result of the disclosure. The specific justification for contacting a collateral source when the patient refuses consent should be documented in the medical record. In this case, making the collateral contacts allowed the clinician to confirm that Mark was truthful in his reporting of his history, his lack of suicidal or violent behavior or threats, and that he has multiple protective factors. Engaging the patient in these discussions ultimately allowed for a safety plan to be developed with his mother.

Duty to Warn/Duty to Protect

Prior to discharge, Mark's PES clinician also had to consider the duty to warn Mark's ex-girlfriend, given his threat of violence toward her. The duty to warn/protect doctrine takes root in the California Supreme Court's *Tarasoff I and II* rulings of 1974 and 1976, respectively. A few key points emerged from these cases. First, the protection of the public against unnecessary acts of violence outweighs patient confidentiality. Second, mental health clinicians are in a special position with regard to their patients and have a duty to take action to protect intended victims from violence. While *Tarasoff I* was focused on a clinician's duty to warn an intended victim, *Tarasoff II* broadened this duty to protecting the victim (by, for example, hospitalizing the patient or involving law enforcement). Since the original ruling, there have been countless legislative and legal actions that nuance the mandate based on the jurisdiction of practice. Based on a review by the National Council of State Legislatures, 31 states have mandatory duty to warn/protect laws, 15 have permissive laws, and 4 have no law.[11,12] Clinicians need to familiarize themselves with the specific regulations in their area of practice.

The ethical dilemma between the duty to protect a potential victim from violence and breaching the patient's confidentiality can understandably cause significant distress for clinicians. Thankfully, as in Mark's case, a majority of these questions are resolved through the process of appropriate clinical assessment and treatment planning, without having to take extraordinary action to make a warning or involve law enforcement. A key component of the evaluation in such a case is the violence risk assessment. The clinician should review the context of any threat of violence, violent ideation or intent, preparatory acts, and aborted attempts. One needs to consider both static risk factors as well as dynamic risk factors for violence. Static risk factors include a history of violence, substance use history, family history of violence, military history, male gender, and younger age of first violence. Dynamic risk factors for violence include access to weapons, current psychiatric symptoms and medication adherence, intoxication, psychosocial situation, and social supports.[5] When contemplating decisions about hospitalization, the clinician should consider which of those dynamic risk factors would be modifiable for the patient in the hospital setting. Remember that duty to protect laws do not expect accurate prediction of violence, but rather that the professional carry out a reasonable standard of care in their assessment.[13] Although he admitted to having the violent fantasy, Mark was assessed to have a lower risk of violence, as he lacked intent and a plan. The ongoing substance use, recent relationship stress, and male gender were his primary risk factors for violence. The overall picture was credible for his threat being made impulsively and partly in the context of intoxication that was now resolved.

When patients make specific threats of violence or describe an urge to hurt a specific person outside of the hospital, several actions can be considered. In cases when the increased risk of violence is linked to acute psychotic or mood disorder, hospitalization should be a strong consideration. An example would be a patient who is threatening violence due to a persecutory delusion that someone is trying to hurt them. Once admitted, the inpatient team should continue to track the risk of violence as the underlying pathology is treated. Often by the time of discharge, the active risk of violence has been mitigated to the point that no further specific action related to the duty to protect is required. It can also be helpful to include the patient in a discussion about the duty to warn, as sometimes they may see the recommended hospitalization as a better option than having their confidentiality breached. In other cases, a patient may wish to give the warning themselves in the presence of the clinician.

If through the PES evaluation, it is determined that the patient is engaged in the treatment process and is safe enough to be discharged, one can work with the patient on an appropriate safety plan. Such a plan can include increased frequency or earlier outpatient appointments, interim safety assessments or bridging services by the mobile crisis unit, enhanced social supports, reviewing coping techniques, and outlining professional crisis resources. Based on Mark's violence risk assessment, and his agreement to engage in clinical services and the discussed safety plan, the clinician was on firm ground discharging him from a duty to protect perspective.

A challenging scenario can arise when a patient threatens violence but does not show signs of an acute and treatable mental illness. For example, a patient who is threatening violence for secondary gain reasons related to gaining admission to the hospital. Often through careful assessment and observation, coupled with review of records and speaking with collateral sources, one can assess the threat to not be credible and appropriately discharge the patient, particularly if it is a vague and non-specific threat of violence. However, if there is a specific target of the threat, this may be an instance when one attempts to warn that person who is being threatened. If contact information is available and the clinician is able to speak with the target of a threat, the person can be counseled about options such as filing a police report or obtaining an order of protection.

Finally, when there is a credible threat by a patient who may be discharged, one can consider notifying the local police precinct or the precinct in the area of the target. One can expect a wide range of responses from law enforcement based on the jurisdiction and the knowledge of the law enforcement official about such situations. The clinician needs to take into the account the response of law enforcement in making a final decision about appropriate disposition. In overriding confidentiality by speaking with law enforcement or a specific target, the clinician should be careful to reveal only details that directly pertain to the threat and mitigating its risk. Prior to taking extraordinary steps such as contacting law enforcement, one should consider obtaining consultation or reviewing with hospital risk management.

The Interface of the Internet and Social Media with Clinical Decision Making

The ubiquity of the internet and social media has presented PES providers with evolving areas of ethical consideration. That the initial 911 call in Mark's case was made in part due to his posting on a social media site is also an increasingly common reality in emergency psychiatry. The suicide note is increasingly being replaced by the suicide text, email, or social media posting. Practical issues arise in trying to verify the exact contents of those notes, as clinicians are rightfully reluctant to have a text or an email forwarded to their own accounts. Services may consider having a general account or posting site that can be used for this purpose. In many instances, a collateral source describing or reading the content has to suffice. The issue of how online communication styles differ from other written or spoken forms as well as the clinical interpretation of provocative or threatening online material is an interesting area that has not been explored in the psychiatric literature.

Mark's case also raises the issue of using internet searches to discover information about patients. A few authors have considered this area of "patient-targeted googling." Clinton et al. recommend that prior to conducting any online search of a patient, a psychiatrist should weigh "its potential value or risk to the treatment."[14] While using a similar framework in justifying online searches as other breaches of confidentiality makes sense theoretically, the ease of "googling" often makes this an afterthought. Furthermore, the lowered sense of privacy societally through the widespread use of the internet and social media can make careful consideration seem unnatural. Still, patients presenting to the emergency department do not generally expect their doctor to be searching their backgrounds online. Clinicians have to be particularly careful in PES settings to avoid online searches simply for voyeuristic purposes. This is a particular vulnerability with VIP patients or when there may be media involvement in a case. It is not uncommon in the course of conducting an online search to find information that further complicates the assessment. For example, one can discover law enforcement information related to a patient that is irrelevant to the evaluation. However, once discovered it could complicate discharge and have to be dealt with as a hospital risk management issue.

Baker et al. outline ten potential situations that may justify patient-targeted googling, including the need to recontact patients about a potential harm, concerns about suicidality, as well as scenarios in which there is concern about patients misusing medical treatment.[15] In Mark's case the concern about imminent risk and the absence of collateral contacts justified the use of a very specific online search to find the necessary contact information for his friend. Informing the patient in advance about the search is preferable if possible. This can also be helpful in the event that other pertinent information is discovered in the course of the online search.

Finally, it is important to document the justification for the search and the relevant information discovered in the same way as material from other sources.

REFERENCES

1. Flomenbaum N, Goldfrank L, Howland MA, Hoffman R, Lewin N, Nelson L. (eds.). *Goldfrank's Toxicologic Emergencies*, 8th ed. New York: McGraw-Hill, 2006, 88–89.
2. Schultz LG. Confidentiality, privilege, and child abuse reporting. *Issues in Child Abuse Accusations, Journal of the Institute for Psychological Therapies* 1990; 2(4). http://www.ipt-forensics.com/journal/volume2/j2_4_5.htm
3. A Guide for Mandated Reporters in Recognizing and Reporting Child Abuse and Neglect. Commonwealth of Virginia Department of Social Services Child Protective Services. Retrieved May 28, 2015. http://www.dss.virginia.gov/files/division/dfs/mandated_reporters/cps/resources_guidance/B032-02-0280-00-eng.pdf
4. Behnke S, Kinscheroff R. Ethics rounds. American Psychological Association Monitor on Psychology May 2002; 33(5). http://www.apa.org/monitor/may02/ethics.aspx
5. Riba M, Ravindrath D. *Clinical Manual of Emergency Psychiatry*. Washington, DC: American Psychiatric Publishing, 2010, 65–68, 261–269.
6. Testa M, and West SG. Civil commitment in the United States. *Psychiatry (Edgmont)* 2010; 7(10): 30.
7. Appelbaum PS. Almost a revolution: An international perspective on the law of involuntary commitment. *Journal of the American Academy of Psychiatry and the Law Online* 1997; 25 (2): 135–147.
8. Christensen MD, Richard C. involuntary psychiatric hospitalization and risk management: The ethical considerations. *Jefferson Journal of Psychiatry* 2011; 11(2): 42–47.
9. Appelbaum PS. The New Preventive Detention: Psychiatry's Problematic Responsibility for the Control of Violence. *American Journal of Psychiatry* 1988; 145(77): 785.
10. HIPAA Privacy Rule and Sharing Information Related to Mental Health (45 CFR164.512. US Department of Health and Human Services. Retrieved June 12, 2015. http://www.hhs.gov/ocr/privacy/hipaa/understanding/special/mhguidance.html
11. Mental Health Professionals Duty to Warn. Retrieved June 24, 2015. http://www.ncsl.org/research/health/mental-health-professionals-duty-to-warn.aspx
12. Edwards GS. Database of State *Tarasoff* Laws (February 11, 2010). Retrieved June 24, 2015. http://www.researchgate.net/publication/228141862_Database_of_State_Tarasoff_Laws.
13. Watson C. The duty to warn/protect doctrine and its application in Pennsylvania. *Jefferson Journal of Psychiatry* 2005; 19(1): 13–18.
14. Clinton BK, Silverman BC, Brendel DH. Patient-targeted googling: the ethics of searching online for patient information. *Harvard Review of Psychiatry* Mar-Apr 2010; 18(2): 103–112.
15. Baker MJ, George DR, Kauffman GLJr. Navigating the Google blind spot: An emerging need for professional guidelines to address patient-targeted googling. *Journal of General Internal Medicine.* Jan 2015; 30(1): 6–7.

12

Evaluating and Treating the Forensic Patient

JENNIFER A. MATHUR, WIKTORIA BIELSKA,
REBECCA LEWIS, AND BIPIN SUBEDI ■

CASE 1: THE PATIENT IN POLICE CUSTODY

History of Present Illness: A 30-year-old man with a psychiatric diagnosis of schizophrenia, multiple prior psychiatric hospitalizations, and arrests for minor offenses presented to the emergency department in police custody for a psychiatric evaluation.

He was found by the police sleeping in the stairwell of an apartment building, and was arrested and charged with trespassing. During the arrest, the patient was noted by police to be mumbling to himself, so the patient was brought for a psychiatric evaluation immediately after arrest but prior to arraignment. On interview, the patient was malodorous and disheveled. He was minimally engaged in the interview and answered most questions with one-word answers. The patient said that he was arrested for "sleeping." He denied having a psychiatric illness and taking any medications, and he claimed that prior hospitalizations were "misunderstandings." He denied suicidal and violent ideation, denied hallucinations, and did not appear distracted during the evaluation. He requested to leave the hospital as soon as possible.

Past Psychiatric History: Although the patient denied a history of psychiatric illness, the electronic medical record revealed a diagnosis of schizophrenia. The patient had been hospitalized twice for symptoms of psychosis. Prior to the first hospitalization, the patient was yelling at people on the street and was brought to the emergency department by ambulance after a bystander called 911. Prior to the second hospitalization, the patient was residing at a shelter and became agitated and verbally threatening when he believed that his clothes were stolen. After both of those hospitalizations, he had not followed up with outpatient treatment recommendations. The patient had a history of arrest for minor offenses, such as theft of service (for boarding a subway train without paying the fare) and multiple prior arrests for trespassing. He had no known history of physical violence, self-injury, or suicide attempts.

Medical History: The patient denied medical problems.

Substance Use History: No reported alcohol, substance, and nicotine use.

Social/Developmental History: The patient was homeless, preferring to live on the streets rather than in shelters. He was single, had no children, and was unemployed. While hospital records indicated that the patient was encouraged to apply for Social Security benefits and Medicaid, the patient denied receiving any benefits or having health insurance.

Laboratory Studies: The patient declined routine laboratory tests, explaining that he wanted to leave the hospital as soon as possible.

Learning Point: Will the Psychiatric Evaluation Affect the Patient's Criminal Case?

When a patient presents in police custody for an emergent psychiatric evaluation for the purposes of determining if immediate treatment is required, the evaluation is not "forensic" in nature. The evaluation is not to determine whether a patient has the capacity to proceed with his legal case, to evaluate if the patient understood his behaviors leading to arrest, or to elicit a confession from the patient. This evaluation is meant to consider whether clinically the patient should be hospitalized or should be given medication in the emergency department. Psychiatrists should remind themselves that they work on behalf of the patient, not as agents of the police department.

However, there are some unique circumstances to consider about patients presenting in police custody who have not yet been remanded to a jail setting. This patient is presenting to the emergency department after arrest but before arraignment. While laws about arraignment vary by state, generally, if the patient does not already have an attorney, the patient will be assigned an attorney at arraignment. At arraignment, the patient will see a judge, be informed of the exact charges against him, and a decision will be made to assign bail, remand to jail, or release him with instructions to return on his next court date. Holding a patient in the hospital for longer than necessary can potentially delay the patient proceeding to arraignment, and therefore delay all of these processes—most crucially, delaying access to legal representation.[1]

To Admit or Not to Admit?

Disposition: The patient declined voluntary hospitalization and repeatedly requested to leave the hospital so that he could "go see the judge." Unlike his previous presentations, the patient was not yelling or threatening anyone. He exhibited poor insight into illness, but remained in behavioral control and had no known history of physical violence or self-injury. Since he did not exhibit signs of imminent dangerousness to self or others, the patient did not meet criteria for involuntary commitment and was released into police custody. Given his history of many prior violations and misdemeanor offenses, and given his history of missing court dates when he was released into the community, bail was denied at arraignment and the patient was sent to the local jail.

CASE 2: THE PATIENT REFERRED FROM JAIL

History of Present Illness: A 29-year-old man with a history of schizophrenia and cocaine use disorder was referred to the emergency department by the local jail for evaluation of suicidal ideation.

On interview, he was vague when describing his suicidal thoughts, failed to state any plan he has considered, and gave conflicting answers about when his suicidal thoughts started. Despite his report of suicidal thoughts, he felt positive about his current criminal case and readily engaged in a conversation about his plans to "get a program," which he said he had already discussed with his lawyer. The patient denied auditory or visual hallucinations, denied sleep or appetite disturbance, and denied any drug use while in jail. His thought process was linear and logical. He reported feeling "very depressed" and that he was being "targeted" by jail officers, explaining that he was angry with a particular jail officer for limiting his time in the library, which was where he liked to research information pertaining to his court case. He proudly said they "had words," but preferred not to talk about it further. He then demanded admission to the hospital, threatening, "Or I'll kill myself."

According to accompanying documentation from the jail unit where the patient was housed, he was to be transferred to a different housing unit for punitive segregation related to assaulting a jail officer. The documentation also indicated he had been compliant with a long-acting injectable antipsychotic medication and that he had been bathing regularly and eating his meals.

Past Psychiatric History: The patient had multiple prior presentations for evaluations of suicidal statements but had no history of suicide attempts or self-harm. He did, however, have a history of two psychiatric hospitalizations for symptoms of psychosis, including gross thought disorganization and poor self-care. His symptoms were effectively treated with antipsychotic medication, which was continued in the jail setting. He had a significant history of violence in the community, against other inmates, and against jail officers. Further, the patient had a long history of arrests for criminal possession of controlled substance, assault, and robbery.

Medical History: He had no history of medical problems.

Substance Use History: The patient had a long history of cocaine dependence but has not used any drugs since his incarceration a few months ago.

Social/Developmental History: The patient was homeless, had never been married, had no children, and had no contact with his family. He spent much of his adult life in jails and prisons.

Laboratory Studies: None were completed.

To Admit or Not to Admit?

He had a known history of schizophrenia, and his history of low functioning and successful treatment of symptoms with antipsychotic medication support the diagnosis. But on exam, there was no evidence of active psychosis, and the patient was known to be compliant with antipsychotic medication in jail. Also, the patient's risk for suicide was assessed as relatively low based on an absence of any history of suicide attempts, as well as his future-oriented thinking despite his reported suicidal thoughts. There was also suspicion based on the circumstances of his presentation that he was attempting to avoid punitive segregation by seeking hospital admission.

Disposition: The patient was sent back to jail with recommendations to continue his antipsychotic medication and be provided with supportive therapy.

Learning Point: Will the Psychiatric Evaluation Affect the Patient's Criminal Case?

In this case the patient is already past arraignment, he has legal counsel assigned, and is awaiting a final disposition of his legal case, he is not expected to be released to the community imminently. The evaluation is for the purposes of determining if he requires acute hospital-level care, not whether he would benefit from treatment in the community or he is fit to participate in a trial. Clinicians who evaluate patients in any kind of custody should be aware, however, that their records and notes could be subpoenaed and therefore should actively avoid discussion of the nature of the charges or documenting any admissions of guilt or assertions of innocence.

CASE 3: ARRESTING A PATIENT IN THE EMERGENCY DEPARTMENT

History of Present Illness: A 37-year-old, single, unemployed man who lives with his mother in a nearby state, with a history of schizophrenia and mild intellectual disability with past psychiatric hospitalizations, walked into the emergency department reporting perceptual disturbances and suicidal ideation. While waiting to be interviewed, he was pacing and banged on the windows, demanding to leave while cursing. With conversation, he was able to calm down on his own and sat quietly waiting to be interviewed.

On interview, he was a poor historian, at times not providing an accurate narrative due to cognitive limitations and disorganization, thus limited information was obtained. He initially denied psychiatric treatment but then admitted he had recently been discharged from a hospital in another state. Upon discharge he had stopped his psychotropic medications but returned to his mother's home. However, he said that morning he decided he no longer wanted to live with her, though could not provide any reason. He said he chose to come to a different state to live in a shelter, so impulsively he took a bus across state lines. He then became scared by the voices he was hearing to kill himself and others, as well as by being alone in the city, thus leading to the current presentation.

At the end of the interview, he refused to get up from the chair, looking down with his arms crossed. After 10 minutes of coaxing with staff presence, he was escorted out of the interview room and into the unit. He then punched the nursing station window and began to bang his arms on the unit windows. He did not respond to verbal redirection and required emergency medication and restraints.

After some sedation, the restraints were removed and he remained calm for a period of time. A few hours later, he became agitated again, responding to internal stimuli, kicking the wall, screaming, and repeatedly trying to enter the nursing station, ultimately, punching a nurse in the face. He again required emergency medication with mechanical restraint.

Collateral information was obtained from the patient's mother and from clinicians at another hospital. His history of schizophrenia with cognitive limitations was confirmed, as was his recent 3-day hospitalization at another facility, where he initially presented as quite agitated, disorganized, and combative, with improvement with antipsychotic and mood stabilizing medication. On discharge, he returned to his mother's house and was scheduled for an interview at a day program the next day, but when told this by his mother he impulsively fled across state lines without taking his medications.

Past Psychiatric History: The patient had a long history of treatment beginning in adolescence and extending into adulthood, including inpatient and outpatient hospitalizations and residential treatment. His history was notable for aggression, including punching and breaking objects, physical altercations, and one instance of putting a knife to his neck but without self-injury. More recently, he was living in a group home for two years but due to concerns about poor treatment; his mother removed him to live with her a year prior. But in that time, he had subsequent hospitalizations, including the one already noted.

Medical History: Diabetes and hypothyroidism but no major past hospitalizations.

Substance Use History: No reported alcohol, substance, and nicotine use.

Social/Developmental History: He was raised by his mother, for the most part living with her throughout his life. He was in special education classes, though graduated high school. He was never married, had no children, and never worked. He had past arrests for assault, including serving 2 incarcerations, the longest being 5 years.

Laboratory Studies: Laboratory results were notable only for elevated non-fasting glucose of 154, and urine toxicology was negative.

To Admit or Not to Admit?

Admission criteria vary across states, as do clinical opinions about whether this patient met criteria for involuntary psychiatric hospitalization. One could argue that the patient was at baseline. He struggled from chronic impairment with impulse control, insight, and judgment, given his intellectual disabilities. He had a long history of aggression and violence both in the community and in the hospital, and an additional hospitalization might not mitigate that behavior. On the other hand, he was at an elevated risk for acute aggression. Though not intoxicated, he had been medication noncompliant for a period of time with command auditory hallucinations to hurt himself and others. While the acuity of an emergency department setting and an inpatient unit could actually worsen his behavior, he clearly had impaired frustration tolerance, and hospitalization could provide structure and consistent treatment.

Disposition: Given the patient's reported symptoms with medication noncompliance, information obtained from collateral sources, and the patient requiring emergency medication and restraint after being interviewed, he was involuntarily admitted to the hospital. As per the legal standard, he presented with a mental illness and as an acute danger to self and others.

To Arrest or Not to Arrest?

After the decision was made to admit the patient to the hospital, he struck a nurse. Although charges vary across states, assaulting a nurse at this location was a felony offense. The nurse had the right to press charges against someone, including a patient, if there was evidence he or she was a victim of an assault. In this particular state, the charge will automatically be the higher felony charge. In this instance, the nurse was punched in the face, resulting in physical and emotional damages, thus the patient could be arrested. However, one could argue that the patient was acutely symptomatic at the time, hearing command auditory hallucinations to hurt others. In addition, he also met criteria for an intellectual disability. Thus, what would be the benefit of arresting an acutely psychotic patient with significant cognitive limitations?

Learning Point: Will the Patient's Psychiatric Evaluation Affect His Criminal Case?

Police may or may not take into account the patient's status as a psychiatric inpatient when determining if an arrest is warranted. If the patient is arrested, records involving the patient's hospitalization are likely to become part of his criminal case via subpoena. Whether his mental illness weighs for or against him in determining his eventual judicial disposition depends on many factors. Again, clinicians should document the patient's clinical condition clearly, and they will have to document the assault as it is part of the clinical course. Caring for the patient who has assaulted a fellow staff member can be difficult due to many factors, but focus should remain on the clinical care.

Disposition: This patient was arrested in the emergency department. As he was still under involuntary admission status, given his acute mental illness and dangerousness criteria but under arrest, he was admitted to a forensic psychiatric unit, designed specifically for patients with symptoms of acute mental illness but who were under arrest and in police custody.

DISCUSSION

The United States has a high incarceration rate. In 2013, approximately 1 in 110 US residents were incarcerated in jails or prisons, and by the end of that year, approximately 6.8 million individuals were under the supervision of an adult correctional system.[2] Given the size of this population, it would not be surprising to find an equally large percentage of inmates with mental illness. At one point in 2005, approximately half the population of inmates in federal prison, state prison, and local jails had a mental health problem.[3] Just by this percentage alone, it is highly likely that clinicians will encounter an individual in the correctional system for psychiatric evaluation in the emergency department. As Daniel (2007) noted, "There are more severely and persistently mentally ill in prisons than in all state hospitals in the United States."[4] Knowledge of the criminal justice and correctional systems can contextualize these presentations and help the clinician with diagnosis, risk assessment, and after-care planning. Further, it is imperative to recognize that the stressors for an incarcerated individual can be different from those who are presenting from the community.

In order to be arrested, there must be some degree of evidence that a crime has occurred that allows law enforcement to take the person into custody. There are two types of criminal charges that one can be arrested for. A *misdemeanor* is a lower-level criminal offense that has a maximum sentence of one year. A *felony* is a more serious offense that carries a sentence of over one year. Misdemeanor and felonies are defined by local criminal law and can vary by jurisdiction. An example of a misdemeanor includes trespassing, while a felony includes murder. The severe and persistent mentally ill may be vulnerable to being arrested for minor crimes rather than being taken to the hospital for treatment. This could be driven by difficulties officers have in recognizing symptoms of mental illness and distinguishing psychiatric pathology from the effects of intoxication[5] but could also be due to local law enforcement policy. The first case is perhaps an example of this, as the police had a choice: they could have simply asked the patient to move from the stairwell where he was sleeping. Instead, the police chose to arrest him for trespassing. From the patient's history, this had occurred multiple times in the past and was highly likely to continue happening in the future.

Individuals who are arrested do not have formal charges brought against them until they see a judge at arraignment. During arraignment the individual, also known as the detainee, meets with legal counsel, has an opportunity to plead guilty or innocent, and is formally presented with charges. A judge can choose to dismiss the charges, remand the detainee to jail, or release the individual to the community with or without bail. If the charges are active, then a date is set for the next hearing.

Given that people with mental illness are overrepresented in the criminal justice system, policymakers have considered the possible benefits to *diverting* mentally ill people out of jails and prisons and into mental health and substance abuse treatment programs. Hence the term *diversion programs*, which can be initiated prior to and after arraignment.

There are two main types of diversion programs. The first is *pre-booking or pre-arrest diversion*. In this circumstance, law enforcement avoids charging a mentally ill person with a crime and instead brings the individual to an emergency room or to a mental health clinician for evaluation. This type of diversion will generally be considered when the behavior is nonviolent and appears to be related to mental illness. These programs require police training in dealing with mentally ill individuals. In the first case example, the patient could have been diverted in lieu of arresting him. He was a mentally ill person found sleeping in an area he was not supposed to and appeared to be hallucinating. The police called to the scene recognized that the person was mentally ill and brought him to an emergency room for psychiatric evaluation; they could have encouraged him to seek alternate shelter in lieu of arrest.

The second type of diversion program is *post-booking diversion*. After an individual is arrested and charged with a crime, there are diversion programs available that offer mental health and/or substance abuse treatment as an alternative to incarceration in jail or prison. Post-booking diversion programs are connected in some way to the court system. After an individual is arrested, the defense attorney might recommend to the court that the individual be considered for a diversion program in lieu of a jail sentence. Eligibility for a diversion program is generally based on a diagnosis of mental illness and the type of criminal charge (although some programs will accept felony charges, many will only accept low-level charges). Diversion programs usually include community-based mental health and/or substance abuse treatment. The prosecutor, defense attorney, defendant, and judge all must agree to a diversion plan. The charges may then be deferred with adherence to the treatment plan being a condition of reduced or dismissed charges.

Most post-booking diversion programs are monitored by a specialized court, such as Drug Court or Mental Health Court. Drug Courts monitor individuals with substance use disorders who were arrested for drug-related offense and are participating in a drug treatment program in lieu of incarceration. Mental Health Courts monitor individuals with mental illness who are participating in mental health and/or substance use treatment programs. In both cases, the defendant must agree to the program and successfully comply with the treatment program in order to remain diverted from jail and/or prison.

As noted earlier, at arraignment an individual can be remanded into custody and placed in jail. A *jail* is a detention center operated by a local (city or county) correctional department. A jail houses inmates who are in custody and still in the process of being tried and/or sentenced. Inmates with misdemeanor, as well as those sentenced to a felony and waiting transfer, are housed in jail facilities as well. *Prisons* are managed at the state or federal level and are reserved for those convicted and sentenced to over a year. Unlike jails, which are built to house detainees for a brief time, prisons are structured for long-term incarceration. Jail tends to be a more fluid, unstable environment, as inmates are frequently entering and exiting the system. Many inmates in jail are also under the added stress of not yet knowing the outcome of their criminal case. Prison, on the other hand, is considered to be more "stable," as many inmates are assigned to a particular housing unit for an extended period with the potential for a static peer group and, in some settings, work programs. This allows for the development of personal and clinical relationships that may be harder to cultivate in jail. In addition, many inmates have had an opportunity to process and come to terms with their conviction by the time they enter the prison system.

There are various options for housing in jails and prisons. *General population* (GP or "gen pop") involves the lowest level of observation. Inmates with mental health problems in general population are considered to only require "outpatient" level services. This often includes access to clinicians in a clinic located onsite, if any services are available at all. Jail and prisons have various stages of programming and housing for individuals who require more substantial treatment. Although there are basic standards for treatment outlined by the National Commission on Correctional Health Care (NCCHC) and the American Correctional Association (ACA), it is important to have a general sense of the housing and therapeutic options in your local correctional facility.[6-8] This knowledge can aid in both risk assessment and after-care planning for those discharged from the emergency department.

There is a consensus that the number of incarcerated mentally ill has risen over the last several decades. Factors contributing to this include deinstitutionalization, the development of more restrictive civil commitment criteria, and punitive drug policies. One of the most commonly cited studies indicated that the rate of serious mental illness in New York City and Baltimore jails was 14.5% in males and 31%

for females.[9] A survey of inmates showed nearly half of jail inmates reported some symptom of major depression and mania, while nearly one-quarter reported at least one symptom of psychosis.[3]

Another concern in jails and prisons is suicide. In a survey of 2002 data, suicide was the second leading cause of death in local jails after natural causes, and it was the third leading cause of death in prisons after natural causes and AIDS.[10] However, it is important to understand that suicide rates vary across demographic subgroups of inmates. For example, the same 2002 data showed that males and whites had the highest rate of suicides in jails and that the rate of suicide increased with inmate age. The youngest jail inmates, those under age 18, were the exception, in that they had the highest suicide rate. Importantly, almost half of jail suicides occurred in the first week of custody. In contrast, state prison suicides most often occur after the first year of incarceration. And the majority of suicides in jails and prisons took place within the inmate's cell. It is these specific risks of suicide that should be considered in the second case. The patient was reporting suicidal ideation, and one must be aware how this patient's demographics might affect his risk assessment.

Two other issues are raised by the second case. One is punitive segregation. Punitive segregation, also known as solitary confinement, is one form of correctional punishment. Inmates in segregation spend up to 23 hours a day in single cells. Concern over the detrimental effects of prolonged isolation has led to changes in the way mentally ill inmates are disciplined while in custody. Both the NCCHC and a task force of the American Psychiatric Association (APA) have provided recommendations on how to provide mental health care for inmates with segregation sentences. Although standards vary by state and facility, generally speaking, inmates with severe and persistent mental illness sentenced to solitary confinement are either placed in modified housing and/or are given access to additional out-of-cell activities. In the second case, the patient was reportedly psychiatrically stable with medication but was about to be placed in punitive segregation. One should consider how destabilizing an environment this could be for someone with schizophrenia and whether that destabilization could lead to increased risk for suicide, particularly given his reported suicidal ideation.

The other issue raised by the second case is malingering. *Malingering* is the intentional production of false or grossly exaggerated physical or psychological symptoms, motivated by external incentives such as avoiding military duty, avoiding work, obtaining financial compensation, evading criminal prosecution, or obtaining drugs.[11] DSM-V recommends suspecting malingering when the evaluation is done in a medico-legal context or the patient has a history of antisocial personality disorder (among other considerations).

A clinician who suspects malingering should utilize multiple sources of information, including interviews and collateral sources. In an emergency evaluation of an inmate, collateral sources are not always available, although more often probably underutilized. Collateral information could come in the form of speaking to family, documentation from jail or prison mental health services, and past medical records.[12] A fourth source of information—psychometric testing to specifically look for malingering—is almost never available and often outside the scope of an emergency evaluation. Malingering in the emergency evaluation of an inmate relies on the clinical interview with a careful examination for evidence of inconsistency.

Questions should be carefully phrased to avoid giving clues about the nature of real psychiatric symptoms. Open-ended questions let the patient tell a complete story with few interruptions, allowing the clinician to assess objective signs of illness (i.e., pressured speech, thought disorganization) and to observe inconsistency in the history.

There are five types of inconsistency: (1) inconsistency within the patient's report itself; (2) inconsistency between reported symptoms and observed symptoms; (3) inconsistency in observation of the symptoms (i.e., the patient appears differently to the psychiatrist than to other staff); (4) inconsistency between performance on psychological testing and the patient's reported symptoms; and (5) inconsistency between report of symptoms and how genuine symptoms tend to manifest in genuinely sick people.[13]

Although the DSM-V recommends suspecting malingering in the presence of antisocial personality disorder, this consideration is less relevant in the incarcerated population. In a prison sample of people suspected of malingering, only about half of those identified to be malingering by psychometric testing carried a diagnosis of antisocial personality disorder.[14]

A clinician who recognizes malingering during the interview may feel irritation at being deceived. However, it is important to recognize that malingering can be functional. Patients may be utilizing their best skills to get out of or avoid sometimes terrible situations. For instance, an incarcerated person may be trying to avoid gang retaliation, abuse, or, in the second case presentation, punitive segregation by obtaining hospital admission. From the inmate's perspective, malingering is a rational response to a difficult situation. Furthermore, deception is a normal and ubiquitous social behavior that clinicians and patients engage in. Deceptive behavior does not preclude the presence of serious psychopathology. The presence of malingering should not limit the assessment to only the patient's reported symptoms. From these authors' clinical experiences, it is not uncommon for a patient to feign suicidal thoughts but actually also be psychotic.

The distinction between real versus feigned symptoms is murkier when an inmate engages in actual self-injury. The emergency room clinician must determine whether the behavior was a genuine attempt to die, a behavior to effect some change in environment or obtain attention, a chronic maladaptive coping strategy, a symptom of another mental illness or intellectual disability, or perhaps a combination of some or all of these.[15] By understanding the inmate's intent, while being aware of the larger context of the jail and prison environment and the inmate's diagnosis and history, the evaluating clinician can complete a more accurate assessment and make sound recommendations.

In addition to mental illness, one should also consider the prevalence of intellectual and learning disabilities among prisoners. A review of the literature demonstrates a range in prevalence rates, but there does appear a portion of inmates in the criminal justice setting that meet criteria for borderline intellectual functioning.[16] In order to make such a diagnosis, not only does the individual need to have an IQ in the range of 71–84, but the individual must also have concurrent deficits in adaptive functioning and coping. It is therefore easy to understand how such behaviors could lead to more police involvement and arrest. Further, such behaviors in jails and prisons could lead to presentations in the emergency department. Being able to distinguish the origins of disruptive and maladaptive behaviors, particularly if they stem from acute mental illness versus chronic cognitive limitations, will aid in the understanding of what can be treated by medication and hospitalization and what might not. The patient in the third case probably had chronic difficulties with frustration tolerance and impulse control, leading to aggressive behaviors. Given his history, it was those chronic behaviors that led to his prior and current arrests, all of which were fueled by an underlying mental illness.

Perhaps most challenging for an emergency room clinician is managing a patient who has possibly committed a crime in the emergency department who may face arrest in the course of treatment. The decision to press charges against a patient is a personal and confusing one. As clinicians, our roles are to care for and treat our patients. However, the rates of assaults against emergency department staff are high. In a 2011 survey of attending physicians and residents in 65 randomly selected US Emergency Medicine residency programs, 78% of respondents reported at least one violent act having occurred in the past year within the workplace.[17] And it appears that nurses most often are the targets of aggression.[18] Such levels of violence have led numerous states in the country to make an assault against a nurse a felony charge.

Although the assault described would be considered a felony offense, one should also be aware of the risks of involving police in clinical care. Decisions to arrest or not arrest are made by police. Even if a staff member requests the police to press charges, it is not up to her what the police decide to do. It is important to maintain a separation between the job of the police and the job of the clinical staff, but also provide support to staff who have been victimized. Inviting police into a clinical space may not have the outcome that was initially intended and can potentially traumatize other patients.

Patients who engage in violence are difficult and troubling to treat. If a staff or hospital is considering pressing charges against an aggressive patient, there are many issues to consider. Is this a patient that has presented multiple times before and is disliked by the entire staff, as they find the person frustrating, annoying, manipulative, or help-rejecting? Is an arrest a means to effectively remove the patient, even just temporarily, from the environment so the staff does not need to deal with him or her for a period of time, thus getting a break from the individual? Does the patient make us feel ineffectual as clinicians, as there does not seem to be any improvement despite multiple presentations and hospitalizations? Have we involved police in order to punish the patient for making us feel this way while also removing him from the hospital system and into the correctional system? Are we confused by the patient's diagnosis and in order to rid ourselves of that confusion we simply diagnosis the individual as having antisocial personality disorder and view arrest as the only reasonable "treatment" approach? Do we believe that arrest is the only way for the patient to change inappropriate coping mechanisms and learn from mistakes? There may be a wish that referral to the criminal justice system will be more effective at modifying behavior than the psychiatric system, when in truth the outcome once the patient is referred is impossible to predict or control and may even cause long-term harm. Patients with criminal justice involvement in their history, particularly felony convictions, will only face additional obstacles to obtaining employment and housing once they are released from jail or prison.

The emergency evaluation of people in custody is fraught with nuance. In addition to the usual clinical concerns, consideration needs to be made for the patient's legal rights (as in the first case), the patient's environment and its role in the production of symptoms (as in the second case), and the very difficult questions that arise when patients commit crimes in the emergency room (as in the third case). Often in these assessments the answer is not obvious. Furthermore, there is much outside the clinician's control (i.e., how and why the police arrest people, whether or not someone goes to punitive segregation, etc.). A reasonable guiding principle is to prioritize the patient's best interest. And often, the best solution is found by consulting with colleagues.

Key Clinical Points

- Evaluation of the patient when police are involved or when the patient is in custody requires understanding of the patient's legal status but is generally not "forensic" in nature in the ED setting. Evaluation should focus on need for treatment or admission.
- Clinicians who evaluate patients in custody should familiarize themselves with local facilities and available treatment for their incarcerated patients.
- Evaluating and treating patients who are involved in the criminal justice system can be complicated by systems issues and personal feelings about criminal justice issues.
- Diversion programs can be helpful in providing mental health or substance abuse treatment.
- Patients who commit crimes in the hospital or ED setting may end up having the police involved. The clinician's first duty is to the patient, and decisions regarding arrest are complicated. Hospital leadership or legal departments may help guide clinicians in these complicated settings, and getting clinical supervision can be helpful.

REFERENCES

1. Gray SM, Racine CW, Smith CW, Ford EB. Jail Hospitalization of Prearraignment Patient Arrestees with Mental Illness. *Journal of the American Academy of Psychiatry and Law* 42:75–80, 2014.
2. Glaze LE, Kaeble D. *Correctional Populations in the United States, 2013*. Washington, DC: Bureau of Justice Statistics, December 2014.
3. James DJ, Glaze LE. *Mental Health Problems of Prison and Jail Inmates*. Washington, DC: Bureau of Justice Statistics, September 2006.
4. Daniel AE. Care of the Mentally Ill in Prisons: Challenges and Solutions. *Journal of the American Academy of Psychiatry and Law* 35:4:406–410, 2007.
5. Lamb HR, Weinberger LE, Gross BH. Mentally Ill Persons in the Criminal Justice System: Some Perspectives. *Psychiatric Quarterly* 75:107–126, 2004.
6. National Commission on Correctional Health Care. *Standards for Mental Health Services in Correctional Facilities*. Chicago, IL: NCCHC, 2008.
7. American Correctional Association. *Standards for Adult Correctional Institutions*, 4th ed. Alexandria, VA: ACA, 2003.

8. American Correctional Association. *2014 Standards Supplement*. Alexandria, VA: ACA, 2014.

9. Steadman HJ, Osher FC, Robbins PC, Case B, Samuels S. Prevalence of Serious Mental Illness Among Jail Inmates. *Psychiatric Services* 60:761–765, 2009.

10. Mumola CJ. *Suicide and Homicide in State Prisons and Local Jails*. Washington, DC: Bureau of Justice Statistics, August 2005.

11. American Psychiatric Association (2000). *Diagnostic and Statistical Manual of Mental Disorders: DSM-IV-TR*. Washington, DC: American Psychiatric Association.

12. Halligan P, Bass C. Factitious Disorders and Malingering: Challenges for Clinical Assessment and Management. *Lancet* 383:1422–1432, 2014.

13. Resnick P. Malingering. In Rosner, R. (Ed.), *Principles and Practice of Forensic Psychiatry* (543–554). London: Arnold.

14. Sokolov G, McDermott B. Malingering in a Correctional Setting: The Use of Structured Interview of Reported Symptoms in a Jail Sample. *Behavioral Science and the Law* 27:753–756, 2009.

15. Fagan TJ, Cox J, Helfand SJ, Aufderheide D. Self Injurious Behavior in Correctional Settings. *Journal of Correctional Health Care* 16(1):48–66, 2010.

16. Herrington V. Assessing the Prevalence of Intellectual Disability Among Young Male Prisoners. *Journal of Intellectual Disability Research* 53(5):397–410, 2009.

17. Behnam M, Tillotson RD, Davis SM, Hobbs GR. Violence in the Emergency Department: A National Survey of Emergency Medicine Residents and Attending Physicians. *The Journal of Emergency Medicine* 40(5):565–579, 2011.

18. Crilly J, Chaboyer W, Creedy D. Violence Towards Emergency Department Nurses by Patients. *Accident and Emergency Nursing* 12(2):67–73, 2004.

FURTHER READING

Massaro J. Working with People with Mental Illness Involved in the Criminal Justice System: What Mental Health Service Providers Need to Know, 2nd Edition September 2003/Revised February 2004. Delmar, NY. Technical Assistance and Policy Analysis Center for Jail Diversion.

Goodale G, Callahan L, Steadman HJ. What Can We Say About Mental Health Courts Today? *Psychiatric Services* 64(4):298–300, 2013.

American Psychiatric Association. *Psychiatric Services in Jail and Prisons: A Task Force Report of the American Psychiatric Association* (2nd ed.). Washington, DC: American Psychiatric Association, 2000.

13

Interim Crisis Services

Short-Term Treatment and Mobile Crisis Teams

ADRIA N. ADAMS, CAMILLA LYONS,
AND MADELEINE O'BRIEN ■

CASE 1: THE MOTHER WITH BORDERLINE PERSONALITY DISORDER, SUBSTANCE ABUSE, AND CHRONIC SUICIDAL IDEATION

History of Present Illness: A 45-year-old divorced woman walks into the CPEP complaining of depressed mood, affective dysregulation, and chronic suicidal thoughts. She is self-employed as a sculptor and lives with her 10-year son. She has a history of alcohol and marijuana use. She states that she has recently been researching methods to kill herself but denies intent to act on those thoughts. She recently moved to the area and is currently without a psychiatric provider and without medical insurance. She asks for medication refills and referral to outpatient psychiatric treatment. She reports having few social supports in the area.

Past Psychiatric History: The patient reports a life-long history of depressed mood and affective dysregulation. She describes having "intense" emotions. She also describes chronic suicidal fantasies as means of "comforting" herself. She was previously diagnosed with borderline personality disorder (BPD). She has no history of psychiatric hospitalizations and no reported history of suicide attempts.

Medical History: The patient reports migraine headaches and a history of endometriosis. She is not currently taking any medications apart from ibuprofen as needed for headache.

Social/Developmental History: She is divorced from the father of her son who physically and emotionally abused her during their marriage. Her son's father lives in another state and her son visits him for one week at a time periodically throughout the year and then for two months each summer.

Clinical Findings: On mental status exam she is well-groomed and elegantly dressed. She is cooperative and well-related. Her speech is rapid but not pressured. She reports: "I think about suicide sometimes. . . . for as long as I can remember." Her thought process is linear and logical. She is very focused on being discharged after her initial evaluation such that she could return home in time to pick up her son from school. She is future-oriented. The social worker at her son's school confirms that there is no concern about the patient's ability to adequately and safely parent her son.

To Admit or Not to Admit?

Disposition: The patient has chronic risk factors for suicide but her risk at time of ED presentation is assessed to be at her baseline. Since she denies active suicidal ideation or intent to act on her prior suicidal "fantasies," she is found not to meet criteria for involuntary admission. As such, she is discharged to home with follow-up in the Interim Crisis Clinic (ICC) for close monitoring of suicidality, ongoing risk assessment, and bridging of care to longer-term outpatient services. She is given an appointment for 3 days after the initial ED visit. The discharging psychiatrist also recommends that the Mobile Crisis Unit be sent to visit the patient at home if she misses the initial clinic visit. No medications were started at the time of the initial ED presentation.

Clinical Pearl

The risk management of chronically suicidal patients with BPD is a topic of debate. Hospitalization may result in negative consequences for patients with BPD. Some of these issues include regressed behavior and concerns that admission may reinforce undesired behaviors.[1] Furthermore there is limited evidence to support the efficacy of hospitalization to treat chronic suicidality.[2]

Course of Treatment: The patient attends four weekly visits in the ICC. During that time her diagnosis is further refined and in addition to BPD, she meets criteria for cannabis abuse. She receives supportive therapy, psycho-education about dialectical behavior therapy (DBT), and medication management with a mood stabilizer and low-dose antipsychotic to target affective dysregulation, anxious rumination, and insomnia. During the course of her treatment, she continues to report suicidal ideation without intent. Despite efforts to reduce substance abuse, she continues to use marijuana daily. She lacks motivation for change. Additional collateral information is obtained from the patient's boyfriend, who denies any concerns about the patient's ability to parent and said she was never seen to be intoxicated in front of her son. He is supportive of treatment and provides helpful collateral to further assess the patient's functioning, aiding in our ongoing assessment of the patient's risk. The patient is ambivalent about psychotherapy, but ultimately agrees to a referral to an outpatient clinic. Unfortunately, there is a long waiting list at a local DBT program, and she continues to require close follow-up during that process.

In the weeks leading up to her son's annual trip to spend the summer months visiting his father out-of-state, the patient becomes increasingly affectively dysregulated and depressed. She experiences difficulties in her work as a sculptor, and she is unable to pay her bills as a result. Her suicidal ideation increases, insomnia worsens, and substance use increases prior to her son leaving her home. Her suicidal ideation becomes more structured, and she discusses numerous plans to harm herself. However, she continues to deny intent and cites her son as her ongoing reason for living.

The day prior to her son's departure, she participates in safety planning with the treatment team. She agrees to accompany her son to the airport with her friend and then travel with her friend to the ED for a voluntary admission. The patient in fact presents to the ED over the weekend as planned, but during the evaluation she grows increasingly ambivalent, declines the admission, and denies she would act on her suicidal thoughts. She is discharged to home with another ICC visit scheduled for the beginning of the following week.

The patient misses her ICC visit and does not answer calls from the clinician. Her collateral contacts have not heard from her for 3 days. Mobile Crisis Team (MCT) is activated, but on their arrival, she does not answer the door. Police gain entry, and the patient is found awake but intoxicated with a strong smell of marijuana in her apartment. She is brought to the hospital for further evaluation. In CPEP, she admits to standing on her roof the night before, while intoxicated, with a plan to jump. She continues to voice suicidal thoughts with plan to get hit by a car or overdose. The patient is involuntarily admitted to the hospital.

Clinical Pearl

The ICC model affords staff immediate and close monitoring of patient based upon their acute needs. In this case, the availability of prompt and close monitoring of the patient in ICC made discharge from the ED on the same day of presentation possible. Many community outpatient clinics do not have appointment availability for such high-risk cases within a matter of days. Another benefit of referral to ICC is the opportunity to refine the patient's diagnosis relatively quickly, to manage acute risk factors, and to begin disposition planning. ICC clinicians have the benefit of frequent, early contact with patients; in this case, that benefit led to the establishment of rapport and subsequently the involvement of her significant others in her care. Communication with collateral contacts helped clinicians asses her current level of functioning and provided additional information regarding any acute changes in risk. It also enhanced the patient's treatment compliance.

As the patient's protective and risk factors were more defined (i.e., her son being a primary factor), deviations from baseline level of risk were more readily obvious to clinicians (without son's presence, her risk of harm to herself increased). In addition, the patient's sudden noncompliance with visits in the setting of recent stressors, along with the collateral information from significant others that the patient has been out of contact, indicated an immediate need to utilize community outreach services, specifically the MCT. The team was then able to assess her risk in the community and bring her to the hospital for admission once her active suicidal thoughts with plan were evaluated.

CASE 2: THE EATING DISORDERED PATIENT
WITH AMBIVALENCE TOWARD TREATMENT

History of Present Illness: A 30-year-old German woman who is a visiting student with no health insurance and a long history of eating disorder is sent to the medical emergency department (ED) from the walk-in clinic for electrolyte abnormality. She had gone to the walk-in clinic the day prior requesting treatment for her eating disorder, which has "spun out of control." She is vomiting after every meal and has been doing so for about one year. She used to induce vomiting but now it occurs "automatically"; she feels the behavior is out of her control. She avoids eating some meals because she wants to stop purging. She feels emotionally and physically "heavy" after consuming a meal. She says she feels better physically after vomiting but worse emotionally. Her mood is depressed. Her Body Mass Index (BMI) is 18.0. Blood work drawn in the clinic shows a serum potassium level of 2.8. She appears shocked to hear there could be fatal outcomes from chronic purging. She is not suicidal and wants treatment.

Past Psychiatric History: The patient was treated briefly for depression after a sexual assault in her late adolescence. She continues to report nightmares and flashbacks of the traumatic event.

Medical History: The patient reports that her menstrual cycle is irregular and that she can go months without having a period.

Social/Developmental History: The patient was born and raised in Germany. She is college-educated. She is pursuing graduate studies in Fine Arts in the United States at the time of presentation.

Clinical Findings/Laboratory Studies: Her heart rate ranges from 37 to 60, with low normal blood pressure. EKG shows sinus bradycardia. Serum potassium level is 2.8. Height is 5 feet, 9 inches. Weight is 122 pounds. BMI is 18.0.

To Admit or Not to Admit?

Disposition: The patient's serum potassium is repleted and she receives intravenous fluids in the ED. A psychiatric consult is requested to evaluate for inpatient admission. The patient declines inpatient psychiatric admission as she does not wish to interrupt her studies. She is prescribed oral potassium supplements, and she is referred to the ICC for monitoring, stabilization, and referral to follow-up care.

Clinical Pearl

While all involved her care to this point wanted her to be treated as an inpatient, the patient did not agree and she did not meet criteria for involuntary admission. Furthermore, she stated she wanted treatment, but she also had very limited insight into the serious potential consequences of her disorder. At this point in time, there was no significant therapeutic alliance between the patient and the providers because she was a new patient. In clinical situations such as this one, there is an opportunity to try to enhance a patient's motivation for change through psycho-education and therapeutic alliance building.

Treatment Course: The patient attends three weekly visits in the ICC. On the first session, she reports continued purging behavior after each meal. She now understands that her low potassium puts her at increased risk of heart attack and death. She reports that her mood is less depressed since she was seen in the ED. She endorses sleeping only 3–4 hours per night. She reports low energy and poor concentration. She reports passive suicidal thoughts but denies any suicidal plan or intent. She says her religious beliefs and her sense of responsibility to her family would prevent her from acting on her suicidal thoughts.

At the end of the first session, treatment with SSRI is recommended and risks, benefits, and potential side effects are discussed. The patient declines medication due to her fear of side effects, specifically her false belief that she will develop tolerance and withdrawal. She is again offered inpatient admission, and she again declines it in favor of outpatient treatment. She continues to voice a desire to get treatment for eating disorder and a wish to stop purging behavior. Her serum potassium level is now 3.5 and she agrees to continue oral potassium supplements. She is referred to the Primary Care Clinic for follow up. An application for Emergency Medicaid is completed.

At the second visit to the ICC, the patient agrees to a voluntary inpatient admission after she makes personal arrangements, including taking a leave of absence from her studies and pending insurance application. She attends her appointment in the medical clinic; the primary care doctor rechecks a basic metabolic panel, which is normal, and counsels the patient the stay hydrated, continue oral potassium supplement, and to consider inpatient treatment along with the SSRI trial.

Clinical Pearl

Eating disorders affect one's physical health in a variety of ways, and coordination of care with the patient's primary care doctor is important to safely manage patients with this group of disorders. Specific physical symptoms to monitor for include hypokalemia, hypophosphatemia, hypomagnesemia, renal function, ECG (bradycardia and arrhythmias), metabolic alkalosis, osteopenia, Russell signs, dental caries, enamel erosion, esophageal tears, delayed gastric emptying, and refeeding syndrome. The role of the primary care doctor is to monitor medical safety, including setting a weight limit and/or a minimal potassium level to safely allow for outpatient treatment.[3,4,5]

At the third visit to ICC, the patient expresses ambivalence toward inpatient admission, wishing to delay 1more week so that she may complete more of her studies. She also voices her fears of the unknown—that is, she does not know what to expect of the inpatient experience. She continues to purge on a daily basis. She voices passive suicidal thoughts, expressed as an urge to "disappear," but flatly denies any intent to kill herself. She remains compliant with oral potassium supplement. She states that she is beginning to tolerate some food without purging. She continues to decline SSRI trial due to her fear of being "addicted," despite efforts to dissuade her of this belief.

Clinical Pearl

Patients with anorexia nervosa (AN) have poor cognitive flexibility.[6] Furthermore, AN patients are characterized by perfectionism and obsessional personality traits. Neuropsychological studies have found impaired cognitive set-shifting and impaired behavioral response-shifting in AN patients, independent of nutritional status and body weight.[7] Traits such as perfectionism, cognitive inflexibility, and negative affect are likely to have a genetic underpinning and may affect treatment resistance.[8] In this case, the patient's inability to incorporate additional information, about SSRIs and their lack of addictive properties and her subsequent refusal of treatment with an SSRI, is an example of how her cognitive inflexibility affected her amenability to treatment. It is important for clinicians to remain in a non-judgmental stance—viewing this behavior as an expected feature of the disorder, rather than a willful or oppositional response to the provider.

The following week the patient presents to the ED to request a voluntary psychiatric admission as planned. She is admitted to the psychiatric unit, where she engages in cognitive behavioral therapy for her eating disorder. On discharge she is able to be referred directly to an eating disorder–focused outpatient program that accepts her insurance plan.

CASE 3: THE WIDOWER SLEEPING IN HIS CAR

Background: The patient is an 85-year-old man who is widowed, retired, and a veteran of the US Navy who has lived in his rent-controlled Manhattan apartment for the past 38 years. He has been referred to the MCT four times previously over the past 10 years for paranoia, turning off the heat in his apartment, keeping his windows wide open and the apartment door propped open when he is home, and reports by building management that he might be sleeping in his car in the building's garage at night. Each time he was seen he was clearly very paranoid, cognitively keen, and physically robust, and he vehemently denied sleeping in his car. He refused all mental health or senior citizen referrals and took great pride in his physical prowess and mental acumen; his case was closed. Patient had also been referred to Adult Protective Services, who deemed him to be delusional but not a danger to himself. He was referred back to the MCT for linkage to mental health services.

The MCT is familiar with the patient from prior visits and reviewed his old charts prior to making their initial visit. The patient had a long history of difficulties with the building management and believed that the executives of the large building management firm have been spearheading a campaign of harassment against him for over 10 years, including stealing from him, failing to make a needed repair in his apartment wall, and constantly pumping toxic fumes through the air vents into his apartment in an effort to oust him from his rent-controlled apartment to procure a much higher rental income. He believed that he is not the only victim of such harassment in the building but felt that he was being harassed the most. Furthermore, he believed that certain city agencies have been colluding with the building management to force him to move out. He turned off all the heat and air conditioning to his apartment to reduce the toxic fumes and he has generally kept all the windows wide open and the door propped open again when he is home to reduce the risk of toxic exposure. On past visits, he was found to spend his time in a rather bare living room with a well-lit table situated strategically between the windows and the door to the apartment. There were piles and piles of papers on the table related to the written complaints about the building management that he had sent to myriad lawyers, politicians, and city agencies. When he leaves the apartment, he packs up all of these papers and other valued items into two large wheeled suitcases that he takes wherever he goes to prevent their theft by the building management.

Current Referral: It is January and bitterly cold. This time the building management had video recordings of the patient's sleeping in his car with the engine running. They also had videos of him refusing to leave the garage and go up to his apartment when the garage attendant asked him to do so. On another occasion, the parking garage attendant had called 911. The patient had been sound asleep in his running car hunched over his steering wheel in the wee hours of a brutally cold night. It had taken several loud thumps on the window to awaken him. He had very begrudgingly gotten out of the car when the police demanded it and had gone to his apartment, only to return to the car the following night. Given that he is in a closed garage, there was concern not only for carbon monoxide poisoning but also for his freezing to death in the car.

Clinical Presentation on Home Visit: The patient permits the team access to his apartment. He shares his fixed persecutory delusional system about the building management but does not appear depressed or manic; he denies hearing voices and does not meet criteria for dementia on brief cognitive screen. In fact, he is quite mentally and physically fit for his age and takes great pride in his daily exercise routine, his volunteer work, his organic healthy diet, and his refusal to be pushed out of his apartment by anyone. He states emphatically that he would see the situation to its end in a court of law and that he would most undoubtedly be the victor. He takes great umbrage about being asked about sleeping in his car and once again adamantly denies that he slept in his car in the parking garage on recent freezing cold nights. When told that the parking attendant had video of his so doing, he states that he maybe had just driven a long distance and was just taking a catnap before going up to his apartment. He points out that he was not breaking any laws.

Clinical Tip

The criteria to remove someone involuntarily from their home for a psychiatric evaluation vary by state. While in New York State clinicians can be licensed to authorize a removal after additional training, emergency medical services and police would be required to carry out a removal, and they may have their own opinions about whether removal and use of force is warranted. In this case, the patient was not removed immediately at this visit, in part because he appeared healthy and it seemed possible that he would physically resist removal, thereby potentially causing more immediate harm.

Clinical Course and Outcome: After much debate among team members and several consultations with colleagues and NYC DMH Crisis Intervention about whether or not patient met legal criteria for removal, the patient is removed to the

ED for a medical and psychiatric evaluation. He physically cooperates with removal, although he objects strongly. He is transported to the ED and after evaluation by ED psychiatrists involuntarily admitted to an inpatient unit, primarily due to video evidence of him sleeping outdoors and concern over acute weather conditions and carbon monoxide poisoning.

The patient contests his admission and is taken to court by the inpatient team, who are able to both retain him in the hospital and obtain a court order for inpatient medication. He eventually agrees to take a low dose of medication that does little to allay his paranoia but does seem to help him to be a bit less intense and more contemplative, he is discharged to the ICC and then moved on the Outpatient Mental Health Clinic and attends, albeit sporadically, for several months. He does not continue on the medication for long.

Outcome: The patient remains irate about his involuntary hospitalization and for many months this only intensifies his paranoia regarding the building management, Bellevue, and other agencies and leads to a letter-writing campaign again, as could be anticipated.

However, as a result of his hospitalization he also resumes contact with his estranged son and considers moving closer to him where he would be able to have family support. He does not resume sleeping in his garage. He is able to have a meeting with building staff where they expressed concern over his well-being, and he is able to accept their concern. While he never develops insight into the essence of his delusion, his interest in writing multiple complaints wanes, and he is able to establish a less contentious relationship with the management. No further referrals were initiated.

DISCUSSION

In systems of care where there is a consistently high volume of patients requiring mental health services, one approach that has been developed to divert patients from inpatient care is a comprehensive crisis service that provides short-term outpatient stabilization, direct linkage to ongoing outpatient services and outreach services such as MCTs. Particularly in areas where there is a long wait for outpatient psychiatric care, short-term crisis bridging services can be extremely useful, particularly in managing high-risk patients. The period following an ED visit is a vulnerable period for patients. More often than not the crisis prompting the visit is not fully resolved. They may not have adequate follow up treatment in place. Clinicians who made the referral to the ED may have decided the patients are "too high-risk" for their practice. Or the outpatient appointment following the ED visit may be for intake evaluation, and there may be a delay in starting treatment. Some psychiatric emergency referrals may suggest that the level of mental health support provided to patients in the community is inadequate.[9] Other factors—including diagnosis, insurance status, socioeconomic status, and race—can limit a patient's access to care during a high-risk period. Referral and successful linkage to appropriate outpatient services from the ED can minimize unnecessary and costly inpatient admissions and reduce repeat ER presentations.

In New York State, the Comprehensive Psychiatric Emergency Program (CPEP) requires availability of "Interim Crisis Services"—including Mobile Crisis—as part of licensing. Various approaches have been taken to meet this requirement, but at Bellevue Hospital's CPEP, the ICC program provides short-term care through continued access to the ED psychiatrist and psychologist, while linking patients to the appropriate services in the community. ICC patients typically are in midst of an acute crisis, either psychiatrically or psychosocially (e.g., housing crisis, rupture in primary relationship, loss of outpatient mental health treatment). It provides high-intensity, easy access to care of limited duration to patients who otherwise might require inpatient hospitalization to stabilize and resolve a time-limited crisis. This service provides close monitoring of chronic high-risk, multi-problem patients but also has the opportunity to transfer patients back to CPEP if there is further exacerbation of symptoms or increase in acute risk factors. In addition, ICC clinicians may also activate a MCT if supportive services or emergency evaluation are determined to be necessary because of missing a visit or other evidence of acute safety or self-care concerns below threshold of calling 911.

MCTs have been in New York for over 40 years but have become increasingly prevalent and structured since the development of the CPEP program. The goals of a MCT are to provide assessment and crisis intervention services for patients who are unable or unwilling to go to an ED or an outpatient provider or who were recently discharged from an ED or CPEP.[10] MCTs have also been used to provide in-home safety assessments, work with police and emergency medical services to assist with crisis situations, and in some states are empowered to involuntarily remove patients from their homes to the hospital for treatment if a threshold of concern for safety is met. In New York State, for example, a clinician working on an MCT can obtain a "removal license" after undergoing additional training about mental health law and crisis management that empowers them to request police and EMS to take a patient involuntarily to a hospital where they are evaluated for admission. Community outreach and "wrap around" services are integral to assure stability, safety, and linkage to recommended outpatient care.

The cases in this chapter examine these challenges and present practical therapeutic approaches for engaging these multi-problem, high-risk patients in treatment during the acute phase following a psychiatric ER visit, or who are referred from the community for safety concerns but are not willing to come to the hospital for treatment. They are also examples of multi-problem, high-risk patients with significant psychopathology. These patients are more likely to evoke strong emotions in treating clinicians, including anxiety and anger.[11] However, with a thoughtful, step-by-step approach, as described in this chapter, these patients can be managed safely. The goal of interim crisis services overall can be summarized as continued assessment bridging to treatment, stabilization, and short-term intensive follow-up. More specifically, key treatment goals of the ICC service include the following:

1. Provide a follow up appointment within five days of the initial ED visit
2. Provide outreach, including telephone calls and mobile crisis visits, for missed Crisis Clinic appointments
3. Obtain further collateral and enlist collaterals for support
4. Refine diagnosis with a keen eye for comorbidity, including substance abuse and personality disorder

5. Stabilize psychiatric symptoms with psychotropic medications and supportive psychotherapy
6. Determine and address barriers to treatment, including lack of insurance or lack of telephone
7. Further assess risk, differentiating chronic from acute risk factors, while managing clinicians' countertransference
8. Determine the appropriate level of care and provide specific resources for follow-up along with "hands-on" help scheduling the initial appointment at outside clinics

The ICC aims to provide prompt follow-up for several reasons: to reassess the patient's safety risk in a timely manner, start treatment quickly, and also improve the likelihood that patients get linked to and comply with outpatient psychiatric follow-up. The rate of patient compliance with referrals to psychiatric follow-up from the ED is usually around 50%.[12,13,14] Wilhelm et al. describe the Green Card Clinic model in Sydney, Australia that aims to provide relevant time-limited intervention and improve compliance with psychiatric follow-up for referrals from the ED by providing an accessible service within a short time-span. Patients seen in the ED for deliberate self-harm are provided with an appointment for the following business day to be seen in their clinic, which provides three visits in total. They found that the initial attendance rate improved.[15]

When patients are not compliant with the initial appointment, they receive a phone call and are offered the opportunity to reschedule. If the referring clinician requested it or if the ICC clinician has additional safety concerns, then a MCT is sent to the patient's home to further evaluate them. There is growing interest in brief interventions for patients who seek evaluation in the ED for attempted suicide and self-harm; these include telephone contacts; emergency or crisis cards; and postcard or letter contacts.[16] Motto and Bostrom found that patients who received letters from staff after they refused follow-up care after inpatient discharge had a significantly lower rate of suicide in the first 2 years postdischarge. Letters simply offered an expression of concern about the patient's well-being and an invitation to respond if the patient wished.[17] Carter et al. partially replicated these findings.[18] Berrouiguet et al. described a study design that would employ SMS text messages to reduce suicide risk among adults discharged after self-harm from emergency services or after a short hospitalization.[19]

After patients attend their first appointment in ICC, the goal is to begin treatment and encourage continued compliance with appointments. Patients accept the treatment recommendations in varying degrees. Motivational interviewing has been identified as a potential way to engage at-risk individuals with treatment and prevent attrition, especially since it allows individual-specific barriers to care to be addressed.[20] Motivational interviewing techniques involve meeting the patient where they are and helping them recognize areas of strength, weakness, and exploration of the patient's perception of their current mental health symptoms as well as willingness to pursue treatment. WHO's global survey of adults found that low perceived need was one of the most significant reasons that individuals did not seek treatment.[21] These results indicate that improving mental health literacy and increasing individuals' knowledge of when it may be appropriate and helpful to seek care may be key approaches to increasing service use rates.

In the first case, the patient's risk to herself fluctuated over time and evolved with her ongoing social context. As the departure of her son became imminent, she became destabilized, her substance use worsened, and she eventually attempted suicide and required inpatient care. Without close follow-up, the patient could have been languishing on a waiting list for care with no one directly responsible for her treatment during this critical period.

Recognizing and reducing barriers to treatment is key in stabilization of these complex multi-problem patients. Individuals often cite structural factors, geographical convenience and availability of care as barriers to service use. For example, among college students at risk for suicide, lack of time and financial resources poses as obstacles to accessing treatment.[22] The WHO's survey found similar structural barriers among adults worldwide, with 15% reporting financial concerns, lack of resources, transportation difficulties, and/or general inconvenience as barriers to help-seeking.[21] It may also be useful to increase awareness about low-cost treatment options (e.g., training clinics or clinics with sliding scale), as well as the range of mental health services covered by one's insurance or institution. College students, for example, may not be aware that their university counseling center offers a limited number of therapy sessions at no cost. Ascertaining Medicaid eligibility and helping patients apply for insurance may also reduce the financial obstacles to accessing care. In the second case, the patient's eating disorder itself posed an obstacle to obtaining care, as specialized eating disorder treatment is difficult to find and many clinicians are wary of taking on such high-risk patients. The patient also lacked financial resources to pay privately for her care. Availability of a hospital-based crisis service where laboratory studies could be obtained and primary care backup is available enabled the patient to have more immediate follow-up both psychiatrically and medically while she transitioned into ongoing care.

Managing high-risk, multi-problem patients during periods of crisis can be complicated. These cases exemplify the importance of diagnostic clarification, a careful and ongoing risk assessment, and determination of treatment needs. A clear understanding of a patient's acute and chronic risk factors as well as mitigating factors should be established. Certain historical factors—including prior self-harm, violence, and substance use—confer a higher level of chronic risk.[23] The factors must be considered when assessing the appropriate level of care and the specific type of services to which the patient will be referred. For example, patients with substance abuse, personality disorder, and/or eating disorder should be referred to specialty clinics with expertise in treating those disorders. Persistent and severely mentally ill patients with psychotic disorders may need intensive outpatient or day treatment. Since these services are frequently not available directly from the ED, a comprehensive crisis service can provide a bridge to the appropriate outpatient treatment services.

Key Clinical Points

- Comprehensive crisis services, including immediate referral to high-intensity outpatient care with capability for community outreach can be used to avoid inpatient hospitalization.

- Patients who require these services are typically challenging in that they have multiple comorbidities, complicated risk, and ongoing psychosocial stressors. Flexibility and coordination of care between services is essential.
- Diagnosis and disposition can be refined and motivation for treatment can be enhanced through short-term intensive follow-up.
- Outreach in the community can be essential in identifying patients who may not otherwise seek care who are at high risk of serious adverse outcomes.

REFERENCES

1. Linehan, M. Cognitive behavioral therapy of borderline personality disorder. New York: Guilford, 1993.
2. Paris, J. Half in love with death, the meaning of chronic suicidality in borderline personality disorder. Harv Rev Psychiatry 2004; 12: 42–48.
3. Currin L, Waller G, Schmidt U. Primary care physicians' knowledge of and attitudes toward the eating disorders: do they affect clinical actions? Int J Eat Disord 2009; 42: 453–458.
4. Mickley D, Hamburg P. Toward optimal health: the experts discuss eating disorders. J Womens Health 2004; 13: 662–667.
5. Sim LA, McAlpine DE, Grothe KB, Himes SM, Cockerill RG, Clark MM. Identification and treatment of eating disorders in the primary care setting. Mayo Clin Proc 2010; 85: 746–751.
6. Tchanturia K, Harrison A, Davies H, Roberts M, Oldershaw A, Nakazato M, Stahl D, Morris R, Schmidt U, Treasure J. Cognitive flexibility and clinical severity in eating disorders. PLoS One 2011; 6: e20462.
7. Friederich HC, Herzog W. Cognitive-behavioral flexibility in anorexia nervosa. Curr Top Behav Neurosci 2011; 6: 111–123.
8. Halmi KA. Perplexities of treatment resistance in eating disorders. BMC Psychiatry 2013; 13: 292.
9. Bruffaerts R, Sabbe M, Demyttenaere K. Effects of patient and health system characteristics on community tenure of discharged psychiatric patients. Psychiatr Serv 2004; 55: 685–690.
10. NYS OMH 2012 Annual Report to the Governor and the Legislature of NYS on Comprehensive Psychiatric Emergency Programs. https://www.omh.ny.gov/omhweb/statistics/cpep_annual_report/2012.pdf. Accessed October 21, 2015.
11. Dressler DM, Prusoff B, Mark H, Shapiro D. Clinician attitudes toward the suicide attempter. J Nerv Ment Dis 1975; 160: 146–155.
12. Blouin A, Perez E, Minoletti A. Compliance to referrals from the psychiatric emergency room. Can J Psychiatry. 1985; 30: 103–106.
13. Dobscha SK, Delucchi K, Young ML. Adherence with referrals for outpatient follow-up from a VA psychiatric emergency room. Community Ment Health J 1999; 35: 451–458.
14. Paykel ES, Hallowell C, Dressler DM, Shapiro DL, Weissman MM. Treatment of suicide attempters. A descriptive study. Arch Gen Psychiatry 1974; 31: 487–491.
15. Wilhelm K, Finch A, Kotze B, Arnold K, McDonald G, Sternhell P, Hudson B. The green card clinic: overview of a brief patient-centred intervention following deliberate self-harm. Australas Psychiatry 2007; 15(1): 35–41.

16. Milner AJ, Carter G, Pirkis J, Robinson J, Spittal MJ. Letters, green cards, telephone calls and postcards: systematic and meta-analytic review of brief contact interventions for reducing self-harm, suicide attempts and suicide. Br J Psychiatry 2015; 206: 184–190.

17. Motto JA, Bostrom AG. A randomized controlled trial of post crisis suicide prevention. Psychiatr Serv 2001; 52: 828–833.

18. Carter GL, Clover K, Whyte IM et al. Postcards from the EDge project: randomised controlled trial of an intervention using postcards to reduce repetition of hospital treated deliberate self poisoning. BMJ 2005; 331: 805–807.

19. Berrouiguet S, Alavi Z, Vaiva G, Courtet P, Baca-García E, Vidailhet P, . . . Walter M. SIAM (Suicide intervention assisted by messages): the development of a post-acute crisis text messaging outreach for suicide prevention. BMC Psychiatry 2014; 14: 294.

20. Britton PC, Patrick H, Wenzel A, Williams GC. Integrating motivational interviewing and self-determination theory with cognitive behavioral therapy to prevent suicide. Cognitive and Behavioral Practice 2011; 18: 16–27.

21. Bruffaerts R, Demyttenaere K, Hwang I, Chiu WT, Sampson N, Kessler RC, . . . Nock MK. Treatment of suicidal people around the world. Br J Psychiatry 2011; 199: 64–70.

22. Czyz EK, Horwitz AG, Eisenberg D, Kramer A, King CA. Self-reported barriers to professional help seeking among college students at elevated risk for suicide. J Am Coll Health 2013; 61: 398–406.

23. Wang Y, Bhaskaran J, Sareen J, Wang J, Spiwak R, Bolton JM. Predictors of future suicide attempts among individuals referred to psychiatric services in the emergency department: a longitudinal study. J Nerv Ment Dis 2015; 203: 507–513.

14

Somatic Symptom Disorders and the Emergency Psychiatrist

LINDSAY GURIN ■

The *somatic symptom and related disorders* category in DSM-5 (renamed from *somatoform disorders* in DSM-IV) can be understood in broad terms as describing patterns of abnormal behavior occurring at the interface of medical and psychiatric illness. The concept of "abnormal illness behaviors," in which patients demonstrate maladaptive modes of experiencing and responding to their own health status and interacting with the medical world, was first proposed by Pilowsky in 1969 as a framework for understanding hysteria and hypochondriasis[1] and remains useful in conceptualizing the psychiatrist's approach to the modern incarnations of these syndromes: factitious disorder; functional neurological symptom or conversion disorder; illness anxiety disorder; and somatic symptom disorder.

CASE 1: MYSTERIOUS HYPOGLYCEMIA

The patient is a 45-year-old divorced woman with no known psychiatric history and with three prior medical admissions for hypoglycemia who is again presenting for evaluation of hypoglycemia. She reports a history of type II diabetes and has been prescribed metformin and glipizide. The last time she was hospitalized, she was taken off of her oral hypoglycemics and was found by a nurse to be surreptitiously ingesting them. She was confronted about this behavior and fled the hospital before a psychiatry consult could be obtained. Today, she was brought from a medical clinic by ambulance for a low glucose. She was given oral glucose solution and crackers in the office, and her glucose is now 80. She is referred for medical admission for insulinoma workup. The medical ED attending recognizes her from prior visits and immediately calls psychiatry: "You have to figure out if she's taking those meds again, otherwise we're going to have to do a million dollar workup." The ED attending places the patient on 1 to 1 monitoring to prevent her from eloping prior to the consult.

Clinical Tip

Consciously simulated illnesses are classified as either *factitious disorders* or *malingering* on the basis of the apparent motivation behind the patient's behavior: in factitious disorders, patients consciously feign symptoms to satisfy an unconscious need to assume the "sick role" (*primary gain*), while malingering patients consciously produce symptoms for a conscious external *secondary gain* such as food or shelter.[2]

Further Observation and Follow-up: The patient denies any surreptitious ingestion but appears very blasé about her repeated medical hospitalizations. On psychiatric interview she is pleasant and cheerful. She denies psychiatric complaints and states that she has no interest in mental health treatment. She has a stable apartment, is financially supported by her ex-husband, and the psychiatrist is unable to elicit any potential secondary gains which may be serving as motivation to be hospitalized. Family collaterals are contacted who report a history suspicious for possible borderline or histrionic personality disorder, with multiple similar medical admissions for bizarre or incongruous symptoms that have tended to occur at times when her work or home life is acutely stressful. The family also finds bottles of diabetes medications in the patient's home. She adamantly denies any suicidal intent and denies intentional misuse of her medications, although when the psychiatrist suggests that she may have a difficulty giving herself the care and attention she needs during times of stress, she agrees to this and admits that she may not be as careful with her medication as she should be during these times. Her glucose stabilizes entirely while she is on constant observation and unable to ingest any medications. While she accepts a psychiatric referral on discharge, she ultimately does not follow up.

DISCUSSION

Factitious disorder is challenging to diagnose and even more so to study empirically as patients tend to conceal their contributions to their illnesses and are not often amenable to participating in research studies. Five levels of factitious disorder have been proposed: (1) fictitious history; (2) simulation; (3) exaggeration; (4) aggravation; and (5) self-induction of disease.[3] In practice, patients can present with one or a mixture of these elements. Suspicion may be raised for the diagnosis when inconsistencies are identified between the patient's provided history and physical exam, or between the patient's history and that documented by outside records; by inexplicable laboratory results (e.g., foreign material in biopsy samples or abnormal results from fluid collected in private but not under observation); or by observed behaviors such as tampering with catheters, removing dressings, or, as in this case, intentional medication misuse.[4]

Factitious hypoglycemia as a result of misuse of insulin or insulin secretegogues such as sulfonylureas is a well described in the literature.[5,6] A 1995 review of 23 cases of factitious hypoglycemia identified four recurring themes: (1) history of the patient or patient's spouse working in a health care field or having sulfonylurea-treated diabetes mellitus; (2) "unusual affect" or history of psychiatric illness;

(3) abrupt onset of symptoms without previous occurrence of minor symptoms; and (4) failure to reproduce hypoglycemia by a 24 h fast.[5] There is believed to be a female predominance and the archetypal factitious disorder patient is a female health care worker, a stereotype which has nevertheless been borne out in multiple studies of the topic.[4] Given the difficulties inherent to identifying this patient population reliably, it is likely that the "female health care worker" is one of several subtypes of factitious disorder (albeit its most well recognized one), and that men presenting with the disorder follow a different demographic pattern.[4]

It is essential for the patient's welfare and for appropriate allocation of medical resources that factitious disorder be distinguished both from true medical illness, on the one hand, and from malingering on the other. Potential secondary gains should be elicited if possible. Careful medical evaluation is necessary before attributing physical signs and symptoms to psychiatric illness and the psychiatrist asked to evaluate for factitious disorder should have a clear understanding of the results of the medical workup prior to that point. Once a simulated illness is suspected, attention should be paid in the psychiatric interview to exploring the patient's understanding of the illness in an open-ended, non-confrontational way.

Treatment and Prognosis of Factitious Disorder

While direct confrontation was once a preferred treatment strategy for factitious disorder, it has been more recently suggested that such confrontation only drives patients away to other providers.[7] Eisendrath has emphasized the importance of allowing the patient to give up the factitious symptom without losing face.[7] In this case, the patient fled when confronted directly over her role in producing her own illness. When, however, the clinician was able to make an empathic connection with the patient and present her with an understanding of her illness that allows for it to be driven by psychological factors without implicating her directly, she was able to ally with the clinician and she accepts a psychiatric referral. She ultimately did not follow up after discharge; prognosis is limited in general.

Key Clinical Points

- Once a simulated illness is suspected, careful evaluation of the patient's role in symptom production and of potential primary and secondary gains is needed to distinguish between conversion disorder, factitious disorder, and malingering.
- Factitious illness production must also be differentiated from self-injurious behavior where the primary goal is self injury or suicide, rather than assumption of the sick role.
- While the most frequently recognized presentation of factitious disorder is of a female health care worker, perhaps with preexisting psychiatric illness, this is by no means exclusive.
- The use of 1:1 constant observation is essential in these cases as patients with factitious disorder are at high risk for elopement from the ED.

- While factitious disorder is difficult to treat and tends to have an overall limited prognosis for recovery, ER interactions with these patients can be geared toward introducing the possibility of a psychological component to the illness and suggesting a potentially beneficial role of mental health treatment without direct confrontation.
- Patients with factitious disorders can elicit strong negative reactions from their medical providers, who may feel helpless and stymied by the patient's apparent insistence on sabotaging treatment attempts. The consulting psychiatrist can assist in mitigating the effect this negative countertransference may have on the patient's care by acknowledging the difficult nature of these patients and providing some insight into the psychodynamic processes driving the patient's behavior.

CASE 2: SEIZURE?

The patient is a 35-year-old married female attorney with two children and no significant medical or psychiatric history who is in your hospital's outpatient laboratory awaiting routine bloodwork when she collapses to the ground and begins to shake. The medical response team is called. On initial evaluation, vital signs are as follows: temperature 98.3; heart rate 86; blood pressure 115/75; oxygen saturation 99% on room air. Her eyes are closed and there is ongoing pelvic thrusting with intermittent flapping of both arms and legs that waxes and wanes in intensity. She is able to respond verbally to her name and says, "I don't know what's going on!" By the time she arrives in the ED, she is awake with eyes open and with continued jerking of her arms and legs. She is seen by neurology consult who, able to slow and eventually completely suppress the movements with a deep breathing exercise, diagnoses a "functional disorder" and recommends no further workup. The movements resolve within an hour and she is discharged home.

Initial Discussion

A variety of terms have been used to describe apparently physical disorders occurring without any known medical cause, originating with "hysteria" in the 19th century and followed by "functional," a reference to disordered functioning of a presumed structurally normal nervous system; "nonorganic," a similar term with emphasis on the suspected non-biologic etiology of the problem; "supratentorial," a suggestion that the source of the problem lies above the level of the tentorium cerebelli (and not, as the patient might believe, in an afflicted heart or gastrointestinal tract); "psychosomatic"; "psychogenic"; and most recently, "medically unexplained physical symptoms" (MUPS). When the complaints relate to a voluntary motor or sensory capacity they are labeled *functional neurological symptom disorder* or *conversion disorder*, with this latter term derived from Freud's belief that such deficits represented substitutions of somatic symptoms for repressed ideas.[8] When the complaints are non-neurologic, the syndrome is called *somatic symptom disorder*.

As a psychiatric disorder that presents only infrequently to psychiatrists, conversion disorder often places the non-psychiatrist in the difficult position of making a psychiatric diagnosis indirectly by proving the absence of a medical or neurologic one. For this reason, there has been interest in describing "positive" clinical signs of conversion disorder. These generally hinge upon examination findings that are either internally inconsistent, as in a patient whose paralyzed leg moves when he is distracted; or externally inconsistent with known patterns of neurologic disease, as in a patient whose sensory loss does not follow known dermatomal patterns.[9] "La belle indifference," an inappropriate cheerfulness or lack of concern in the face of apparent significant neurologic deficit, was identified by Freud as suggestive of conversion disorder and has historically been considered a useful clinical sign but has not been validated with empiric studies.[10]

In the literature and in practice, conversion disorders are approached according to which neurologic syndrome they most resemble. Suggested positive clinical signs differ by syndrome. Examples include the Hoover sign for motor conversion disorder, in which patients cannot extend at the hip when tested directly but do involuntarily so when flexing the good leg against resistance; and the "noneconomical" or "astasia-abasia" gait for functional gait disorders, in which the gait movements are eccentric to the center of gravity or otherwise require a degree of motor control and coordination that precludes a true neurologic deficit.[10] A major subclass of conversion disorders, and the one featured in this case, mimics epileptic seizures and has been termed *psychogenic nonepileptic seizures* (PNES). For the specific case of PNES, evidence-based clinical signs suggesting functional disorder include, among others, closed eyes; a fluctuating course; long episode duration; side-to-side head or body movements; memory recall for the period of apparent unconsciousness; and ictal crying.[11] Pelvic thrusting during episodes has historically been associated with PNES but notably is also associated with frontal lobe seizures.[11] The patient's normal vital signs during the episode are also suggestive of a nonepileptic event (seizures tending to be accompanied by sympathetic hyperactivity), as is her ability to continue to communicate throughout the event.

Case Continued

The patient presents again the next morning with her husband who states the patient's movements returned later that night and could not be suppressed with any of the suggested techniques. She has brought her teddy bear with her from home. Psychiatry and neurology are both consulted. On psychiatric interview, she is pleasant and well related. During the course of the interview, she has several two- to three-minute episodes in which her eyes are closed and her arms and legs jerk with waxing and waning frequency and at different frequencies from each other. She is able to answer in a soft voice during these episodes and appears not to be distressed. When the episodes end she returns immediately to what she had been speaking about before the episode. She denies mood symptoms and is most concerned about missing a major work presentation today. Her family history is significant for a younger sister with epilepsy. She tells the psychiatrist she would like to figure out what is causing her movements so she can go home and get back to work.

On the way out of the ED the clinician encounters the consulting neurologist who tells you she thinks the patient's movements are "supratentorial" but that "seizures can trick you" and she is nevertheless going to admit her for video-electroencephalographic (VEEG) monitoring. She asks for the psychiatric impression: "Is she faking? Am I just giving her what she wants if I admit her?"

Further Discussion

The DSM-5 diagnosis criteria for conversion disorder emphasize the discrepancy between clinical findings and known patterns of neurologic or medical disease and specify that the symptoms must cause distress. The requirements that the symptoms not be "feigned" intentionally and that the onset be associated with a known psychological stressor were dropped in the transition from DSM-IV-TR to DSM-5, acknowledging the difficulty of determining these features in many cases. As in all of the somatic symptom disorders, close collaboration between the psychiatrist and the medical diagnostician is essential. In this case, while there are many features suggestive of a functional neurologic disorder, the neurologist is appropriately requesting further, more definitive workup and can be reassured that while doing so may be giving the patient "what she wants" in the immediate short term, she will benefit in the longer term from being appropriately diagnosed. While anecdotally associated with personality disorder, the presence of an age-inappropriate toy (the "Teddy bear sign") has been shown to be associated with the presence of nonepileptic events in patients being admitted electively to epilepsy monitoring units for VEEG monitoring.[12]

Case Conclusion

The patient is admitted to the neurology service for VEEG monitoring. Several typical episodes are captured and EEG is notably normal during those times. The neurology team and the psychiatry consultation-liaison team meet jointly with the patient to discuss the diagnosis of PNES. She is not started on antiepileptic medications. She is scheduled for both neurology and psychiatry follow-up outpatient visits.

Key Clinical Points

- Conversion disorder (functional neurologic symptom disorder) is diagnosed based on history and exam findings that are inconsistent with neurologic patterns of illness.
- An obvious psychosocial stressor is not necessary for diagnosis, nor is proof that the patient is not intentionally feigning (although if there is evidence that the patient is feigning, conversion disorder is excluded).
- As in the case of factitious disorder, the psychiatrist's role as a liaison between patient and primary medical team is of the utmost importance in cases of conversion disorder

CASE 3: THE "FREQUENT FLYER"

The patient is a 55-year-old man with a history of depression and anxiety for which he is not currently in treatment, with medical history of hypertension and diabetes, receiving disability payments for chronic back pain, who is in the ED today for the fifth time this week complaining of vague malaise and multi-system complaints. Earlier this week, he presented with tinnitus and vertigo and received magnetic resonance imaging (MRI) of the brain to rule out acute stroke. Yesterday, he presented with gastrointestinal discomfort and chest pressure and underwent a negative workup for acute coronary syndrome. He is back today reporting that he still does not feel well and he is worried that something is "really wrong." He feels easily fatigued and reports difficulty concentrating. He has been spending most nights reading about his symptoms on the internet instead of sleeping and he is requesting computed tomography (CT) scans of his chest, abdomen and pelvis to exclude cancer. Vital signs are as follows: temperature 98.3; heart rate 96; blood pressure 144/85; oxygen saturation 99% on room air; finger-stick glucose 98. Initial diagnostic studies reveal a normal complete blood count, basic metabolic panel and liver function testing. Electrocardiogram reveals normal sinus rhythm with mild left ventricular hypertrophy. Cardiac troponins are negative. The ED attending requests a psychiatry consult prior to further medical evaluation: "He has real risk factors but I can't find anything wrong. I think this is all from his depression. Am I going to have to rule out ACS every time this guy comes in?"

Initial Discussion

Medically unexplained physical symptoms (MUPS) are physical symptoms for which no medical cause has been found. They are encountered commonly in the primary care and emergency department settings and are estimated to affect 6% of the population and to account for up to half of all consultations in primary care clinics.[13] Patients with MUPS tend to be disproportionately high utilizers of medical resources[14] and to experience increased rates of disability.[15,16] Symptoms can occur singly or in clusters. Chronic fatigue syndrome, fibromyalgia, and irritable bowel syndrome represent the most commonly encountered unexplained symptom clusters but most medical specialties have at least one such syndrome associated with them: in addition to neurology and conversion disorder (discussed in detail in case 2), examples include cardiology and non-cardiac chest pain; otolaryngology and globus; rheumatology and multiple chemical sensitivity; and gynecology and chronic pelvic pain, to name a few.[13] Many patients meet criteria for more than one syndrome, providing support for the possibility of one or several common etiologic factors driving these apparently disparate presentations.[17-19]

While our patient may be said at this point to have MUPS, the leap from MUPS to a psychiatric diagnosis of a mood, anxiety or somatoform disorder requires further information. Perhaps even more so than for the other somatoform disorders, the naming and definition of what is now called *somatic symptom disorder* in DSM-5 has been fraught with controversy. The diagnosis of its DSM-IV predecessor, *somatization disorder,* required the presence of 1) a minimum of eight multisystem complaints; and 2) the medical determination that, after "appropriate investigation," these symptoms were either entirely medically unexplained or were related to a known medical illness but disproportionate in degree of severity. Missing from this formulation is any reference to psychiatric symptoms or psychological distress and critics argued that absence of a medical explanation for an experience was an inadequate criterion on which to diagnose psychiatric illness. DSM-5 explicitly acknowledges this critique and the new category of somatic symptom disorders requires the presence of abnormal or excessive thoughts, feelings or behaviors in response to one or more somatic symptoms, whether or not there is a medical explanation for these symptoms. As in conversion disorder, the emphasis now is on eliciting positive clinical findings to support a psychiatric diagnosis, rather than assigning a "mentally ill" label to any syndrome not clearly diagnosable through available medical techniques.

Case Continued

The patient is irritated that psychiatry has been asked to see him but he reluctantly agrees to participate in an interview. He reports prior diagnoses of depression and anxiety with trials of selective serotonin reuptake inhibitors (SSRIs) in the past but he says that these "never worked" and he stopped them on his own. He has had brief periods of engagement with psychotherapy but says this felt like "a racket" and he never saw any clear benefit. He acknowledges that his mood is "never great" but he denies feeling depressed. He denies a history of trauma. When he is not feeling ill he enjoys going to movies with his girlfriend and spending time with friends. He does note that he has been under significant stress recently as his sister died of lung cancer a year ago and his girlfriend is currently disabled by severe rheumatoid arthritis. He identifies himself as "the healthy one" although he has not been able to work since he injured his back several years ago—in addition to chronic back pain, he experiences migraines, fatigue, and chronic intermittent dizziness which prevent him from returning to his previous job in construction. It emerges that his girlfriend is in fact currently hospitalized at the same hospital to which he has presented, and that his symptoms tend to worsen after he visits her. He admits that it is difficult for him to disclose emotional content to others and that he tends to keep his feelings "bottled up inside" He agrees that he is worried about his girlfriend. While he is able to appreciate the general contribution of psychosocial stress to physical wellbeing and he admits that some of his symptoms (e.g. poor concentration) may be exaggerated by lack of sleep, he resists a fully psychological explanation for his symptoms, saying that he is "not crazy" and "doctors always telling me nothing's wrong is the most stressful thing of all." He nevertheless agrees to "think about" a referral to cognitive-behavioral therapy (CBT) on the suggestion that he might learn strategies for coping with his own and his girlfriend's ongoing medical illness.

Further Discussion

Our patient meets criteria for somatic symptom disorder on the basis of his persistent distress related to, and excessive time and energy expended on, somatic symptoms. Whether or not these symptoms are related to a known medical illness is not relevant to diagnosing somatic symptom disorder but, as our patient points out, the diagnostic uncertainty and repeated invalidation often encountered during the evaluation for medically unexplained symptoms is itself a stressor that can exacerbate symptoms. Suggested etiologies of medically unexplained symptoms generally fall into three broad categories:[18]

1. Response to trauma. Numerous studies have demonstrated a relationship between trauma history—particularly childhood sexual abuse—and subsequent medically unexplained symptoms.[20]
2. Psychiatric illness. MUPS are associated with increased likelihood of comorbid anxiety or depressive disorder[21-23] and in some instances may be related to neurovegetative symptoms of depression or somatic manifestations of anxiety.
3. Disturbed physiologic processes invisible to current medical investigative techniques.

The true explanation for most medically unexplained symptoms is likely some mix of all of these plus other contributors not yet identified. Each of the first two factors, at least, seems to be neither necessary nor sufficient for the development of MUPS as there are patients with MUPS who have neither of these features. Cognitive and perceptual models have increasingly become of interest: Barsky and Wyshak proposed understanding hypochondriacs as "somatosensory amplifiers" who are overly sensitive to benign somatic perceptions and who misattribute these perceptions to illness,[24] while others have suggested a role for impaired filtering of normal body perceptions.[25] A cognitive tendency to catastrophize pain and other bodily sensations may also contribute.[25] Impairments in mental representation of one's own emotions (alexithymia) and the emotions of others (affective theory of mind) have also been associated with MUPS, suggesting, among other things, the possibility of a modern approach to the Freudian construct of coping with difficult emotional experiences by "converting" them into physical ones.[26-28] In all models of unexplained symptoms, there is a growing appreciation for the interaction between physiology, psychology, and social experience that serves to produce and maintain an abnormal and often disabling approach to managing one's own health and illness.

With cognitive distortions in mind as perhaps the most readily treatable aspect of this complex syndrome, cognitive-behavioral therapy (CBT) has become the treatment of choice for MUPS and its efficacy in reducing symptoms, disability, and psychological distress is consistently demonstrated in studies.[29,30] Antidepressants have generally been considered the first-line pharmacologic agents for somatoform disorders. With the caveat that the available evidence is "very low quality," a recent Cochrane review found new-generation antidepressants to be "moderately effective" in treating somatoform disorders and found some evidence that a combination of antidepressants and antipsychotics was more effective than antidepressants alone. The reviewers also suggested that the risks of somatic adverse effects related to these medications, in individuals already focusing on somatic symptoms, may outweigh the benefits of their use in some cases.[31]

Because patients with MUPS are often reluctant to seek psychiatric care, one potentially productive avenue for intervention involves providing indirect psychiatric support via recommendations given to the medical provider. A recent Cochrane review found that use of a psychiatric "consultation letter" in primary care reduced medical costs and improved physical functioning in patients with somatoform disorders.[32] In this intervention, a consulting psychiatrist evaluates the patient and, if a somatoform diagnosis is made, subsequently provides a letter to the primary care provider confirming and explaining the diagnosis of MUPS, specifically including its low risk of mortality. The letter also provides detailed recommendations for communication with the patient and for continued clinical management. Importantly, this intervention involves the patient seeing a psychiatrist only once and continuing to receive care from the primary care provider afterward, minimizing stigma and feelings of abandonment while also providing the medical clinician with necessary support.

Clinical Pearl

The mere fact of having medically unexplained symptoms—even many of them, across multiple organ systems—is no longer enough to qualify a patient for a psychiatric diagnosis. In addition to the negative criterion of no medical etiology being found, there must additionally be some positive clinical finding: this can be a "functional" somatic finding, as in the conversion disordered patient who can move his legs to run but not to walk; or a psychological finding, as in our patient who is so distressed over what his symptoms might portend that he is unable to sleep at night and has put all of his usual activities aside to pursue repeated ED evaluations.

Clinical Pearl

There are three important aspects of interventions for patients with persistent medically unexplained symptoms and somatic symptom disorders:

1. Psychiatric screening to identify and treat psychiatric comorbidities.
2. Structured case management including scheduling regular medical visits and limiting referrals and further diagnostic testing.
3. Attention to physician-patient communication—specifically, taking the patient's complaints seriously, doing a physical examination, not telling the patient "it's all in your head."[32]

Case Conclusion

The patient does not meet full criteria for a major depressive disorder or an anxiety disorder but he does meet criteria for chronic dysthymia. He is not interested in seeing a psychiatrist currently. He likes his primary care provider and tries to see her on an as-needed basis but she is not always able to fit him in urgently when he experiences symptom exacerbations—hence his frequent ED visits. He himself is frustrated by the amount of time he has had to spend in EDs and he agrees that seeing his doctor on a regularly scheduled basis might provide him with the ongoing medical attention he needs and might help to minimize his ED visits. He calls from the ED to schedule his next appointment with her. The psychiatrist also calls the primary care provider to discuss somatic symptom disorder, with an emphasis on the connection the patient already feels to her and the positive role she can play merely by seeing him regularly and listening to his complaints in an nonjudgmental way.

Clinical Pearl

Somatic symptom disorders are best diagnosed and managed within the context of a longitudinal relationship with a medical provider, making them particularly challenging for the ED physicians who encounter them in one-off visits. As in factitious and conversion disorders, direct confrontation tends not to be productive and telling a patient "it's all in your head" or "it's nothing" can fuel frustration and distrust. In this case, the psychiatrist validated the patient's somatic experience and allied with him around the stress of being a caregiver to his girlfriend and his frustration with having to spend so much time in the ED—in this light, he was able to view both CBT and regularly scheduled primary care visits as more acceptable interventions

Final Thoughts

Nowhere in psychiatry is the "liaison" component of consultation-liaison psychiatry more important than in management of somatoform disorders, where frustrations from patients and providers alike over the perceived failure to find a medical diagnosis can tangle together in complex and counterproductive dynamics. While these patients often resist ongoing direct psychiatric treatment, there is evidence that even one-time psychiatric evaluation can be useful in providing diagnostic clarity and supporting the medical clinician's relationship with the patient; while this data is largely from the primary care setting, it is worth keeping in mind in the ED consultation setting. Correctly identifying somatoform disorders (Table 14.1) is crucial both for providing the patient with psychiatric care, if needed, but also for avoiding iatrogenic injury: studies have shown patients with somatic disorders to be more likely to undergo extensive medical and surgical procedures, generally with little benefit.[33,34] While somatoform disorders are chronic and will not be

Table 14.1 QUICK GUIDE TO SOMATOFORM DISORDERS

Diagnosis	Symptom production	Motivation
Malingering	Conscious	Secondary (conscious) gain, e.g. food, shelter, money
Factitious disorder	Conscious	Primary (unconscious) gain, i.e., "sick role," care and attention, socially acceptable relief from responsibilities
Somatic symptom and conversion disorders	Unconscious	Primary (unconscious) gain

cured with a one-time ED psychiatry consult, the ED psychiatrist can aim to provide the patient with a positive mental health treatment encounter and the medical clinicians with helpful management approaches and communicative techniques for interacting with these complex patients.

REFERENCES

1. Pilowsky I. The concept of abnormal illness behavior. Psychosomatics 1990;31:207–313.
2. McCullumsmith CB, Ford CV. Simulated illness: the factitious disorders and malingering. Psychiatric Clinics of North America 2011;34:621–641.
3. Folks D, Feldman M, Ford C. Somatoform disorders, factitious disorders, and malingering. Psychiatric Care of the Medical Patient 2000:459–475.
4. Krahn LE, Hongzhe L, Kevin O'Connor M. Patients who strive to be ill: factitious disorder with physical symptoms. American Journal of Psychiatry 2003;160(6):1163–1168.
5. Klonoff DC, Barrett BJ, Nolte MS, Cohen RM, Wyderski R. Hypoglycemia following inadvertent and factitious sulfonylurea overdosages. Diabetes Care 1995;18:563–567.
6. Scarlett JA, Mako ME, Rubenstein AH, et al. Factitious hypoglycemia: diagnosis by measurement of serum C-peptide immunoreactivity and insulin-binding antibodies. New England Journal of Medicine 1977;297:1029–1032.
7. Eisendrath SJ. Factitious physical disorders: treatment without confrontation. Psychosomatics 1989;30:383–387.
8. Ford CV, Folks DG. Conversion disorders: an overview. Psychosomatics 1985;26:371–383.
9. Daum C, Monica H, Selma A. The value of 'positive' clinical signs for weakness, sensory and gait disorders in conversion disorder: a systematic and narrative review. Journal of Neurology, Neurosurgery & Psychiatry (2013): jnnp-2012.
10. Aybek S, Kanaan RA, David AS. The neuropsychiatry of conversion disorder. Current Opinion in Psychiatry 2008;21:275–280.
11. Avbersek A, Sisodiya S. Does the primary literature provide support for clinical signs used to distinguish psychogenic nonepileptic seizures from epileptic seizures? Journal of Neurology, Neurosurgery & Psychiatry 2010;81:719–725.
12. Burneo J, Martin R, Powell T, et al. Teddy bears: an observational finding in patients with non-epileptic events. Neurology 2003;61:714–715.
13. Stephenson D, Price J. Medically unexplained physical symptoms in emergency medicine. Emergency Medicine Journal 2006;23:595–600.
14. Barsky AJ, Ettner SL, Horsky J, Bates DW. Resource utilization of patients with hypochondriacal health anxiety and somatization. Medical Care 2001;39:705–715.
15. van der Leeuw G, Gerrits M, Terluin B, et al. The association between somatization and disability in primary care patients. Journal of Psychosomatic Research 2015.
16. Rask MT, Rosendal M, Fenger-Grøn M, Bro F, Ørnbøl E, Fink P. Sick leave and work disability in primary care patients with recent-onset multiple medically unexplained symptoms and persistent somatoform disorders: a 10-year follow-up of the FIP study. General Hospital Psychiatry 2015;37:53–59.

17. Burton C. Beyond somatisation: a review of the understanding and treatment of medically unexplained physical symptoms (MUPS). British Journal of General Practice 2003;53:231–239.

18. Aaron LA, Buchwald D. A review of the evidence for overlap among unexplained clinical conditions. Annals of Internal Medicine 2001;134:868–881.

19. Aggarwal VR, McBeth J, Zakrzewska JM, Lunt M, Macfarlane GJ. The epidemiology of chronic syndromes that are frequently unexplained: do they have common associated factors? International Journal of Epidemiology 2006;35:468–476.

20. Roelofs K, Spinhoven P. Trauma and medically unexplained symptoms: towards an integration of cognitive and neuro-biological accounts. Clinical Psychology Review 2007;27:798–820.

21. De Waal MW, Arnold IA, Eekhof JA, Van Hemert AM. Somatoform disorders in general practice. The British Journal of Psychiatry 2004;184:470–476.

22. Steinbrecher N, Koerber S, Frieser D, Hiller W. The prevalence of medically unexplained symptoms in primary care. Psychosomatics 2011;52:263–271.

23. Henningsen P, Zimmermann T, Sattel H. Medically unexplained physical symptoms, anxiety, and depression: a meta-analytic review. Psychosomatic Medicine 2003;65:528–533.

24. Barsky AJ, Wyshak G. Hypochondriasis and somatosensory amplification. The British Journal of Psychiatry 1990;157:404–409.

25. Rief W, Broadbent E. Explaining medically unexplained symptoms-models and mechanisms. Clinical Psychology Review 2007;27:821–841.

26. Kooiman CG. The status of alexithymia as a risk factor in medically unexplained physical symptoms. Comprehensive Psychiatry 1998;39:152–159.

27. De Gucht V, Heiser W. Alexithymia and somatisation: a quantitative review of the literature. Journal of Psychosomatic Research 2003;54:425–434.

28. Stonnington CM, Locke DE, Hsu C-H, Ritenbaugh C, Lane RD. Somatization is associated with deficits in affective theory of mind. Journal of Psychosomatic Research 2013;74:479–485.

29. Kroenke K. Efficacy of treatment for somatoform disorders: a review of randomized controlled trials. Psychosomatic Medicine 2007;69:881–888.

30. Sumathipala A. What is the evidence for the efficacy of treatments for somatoform disorders? A critical review of previous intervention studies. Psychosomatic Medicine 2007;69:889–900.

31. Kleinstäuber M, Witthöft M, Steffanowski A, van Marwijk H, Hiller W, Lambert MJ. Pharmacological interventions for somatoform disorders in adults. Cochrane Database of Systematic Reviews 2014;11.

32. Hoedeman R, Blankenstein AH, van der Feltz-Cornelis CM, Krol B, Stewart R, Groothoff JW. Consultation letters for medically unexplained physical symptoms in primary care. The Cochrane Library 2010.

33. Fink P. Surgery and medical treatment in persistent somatizing patients. Journal of Psychosomatic Research 1992;36:439–447.

34. Kouyanou K, Pither CE, Wessely S. Iatrogenic factors and chronic pain. Psychosomatic Medicine 1997;59:597–604.

15

Psychodynamic Aspects of Emergency Psychiatry

DANIEL J. ZIMMERMAN ■

A mantra of psychodynamic psychiatry is "Don't just do something, sit there." Therefore, psychodynamic theory and methods of treatment may seem far removed from the emergency setting, which is busy, frequently chaotic, and requires rapid decision making and action. However, knowledge of psychodynamic principles can help shape the perceptions and clinical choices of clinicians in many settings, as they offer a way to understand the patient's behavior within the clinical encounter, and help the clinician be aware of his or her own reactions and avoid distorted reactions to difficult patients. At the very least, the psychodynamically-informed emergency room clinician will do a better job of "doing no harm" to some of the most vulnerable patients found in medicine, and, at best, of providing healing, comfort, and hope even in the brief clinical interactions of the emergency room.

The focus of this chapter will be to show through emergency psychiatry case examples how psychodynamic principles like the unconscious, drive, stages of development, projection and displacement, and transference/countertransference (among other concepts, mentioned in italics) can be used to illuminate the clinical situation and influence treatment.

CASE 1: BASICS OF PSYCHODYNAMIC THEORY

A 54-year-old divorced shelter-domiciled man was brought into the emergency room by ambulance. The triage sheet noted a chief complaint of "They took my balls!" Initial brief mental status examination revealed a poorly groomed man outraged to have been brought to the hospital and with an angry, defiant attitude, but he could be verbally redirected and reluctantly complied with intake protocols. Review of the patient's hospital electronic record showed that six weeks prior he had presented to the medical emergency room with a laceration to his scrotum reportedly caused by a dog bite, had received wound care and was given a follow-up appointment with the urologist, which he had missed. One month later (two weeks prior to the current presentation) he had re-presented to the medical emergency room with testicular rupture, for which he was admitted to the hospital for emergent unilateral orchidectomy, and was discharged after 3 days. Today, the ambulance had been called to the shelter because he had gotten into a shouting match with another shelter resident, and when police arrived, he began ranting to police officers about how the doctors had "taken his balls off" without his permission. He was minimally cooperative and not very forthcoming during the interview. He reported a prior psychiatric diagnosis of "bipolar" with hospitalizations in the remote past and was receiving social security disability benefits because of mental illness. He was not on psychiatric medications and had received no recent treatment. He admitted to having had a few beers earlier in the day. He was afebrile with a clear sensorium, was not obviously demented (was able to recall 2/3 objects after 5 minutes and draw a clock accurately), and did not appear currently intoxicated, as confirmed by a negative blood alcohol level (BAL). His affect was angry. He made vengeful threats with paranoid and homicidal content toward the surgeons who had operated on him.

Treatment Issues

Because of homicidal threats, and possible inability to care for self (as he had missed the urology appointment and allowed his physical health to deteriorate), there could have been grounds for involuntary hospitalization to protect the safety of the patient and others. Given his angry affect and lack of recent treatment in addition to the acute medical stressor and chronic stressors of poverty and homelessness, a manic or mixed mood relapse or recurrence was a prominent diagnostic consideration (with a possible role for substance abuse as well). However, he denied other symptoms and signs of a mood episode including depressed mood or euphoria, recent sleep or appetite change, slowing down or speeding up of thoughts, and though he had an angry affect, he did not have pronounced mood lability or grandiosity. Inpatient hospitalization was recommended, but he was not interested in that or any other treatment help. A discussion with him about medical and psychiatric contingencies revealed a sufficient capacity to act in his own rational interest, and when asked if he actually intended to harm the surgeons, he said "the bastards deserved it" but denied having a plan or intent to do so. He was retained in the emergency room overnight. He was able to calm down after discussing his rage and frustration with the evaluating clinician, and was discharged with only a shelter clearance form in the morning, as he again refused any follow-up psychiatric treatment.

Psychodynamic Aspects of the Case

Psychodynamic theory is a set of principles about the structure and function of the developing and adult mind. They describe how the human mind contains conflict because it is made up of separate agencies with different wills, and label as *drive* the psycho-physical force by which the mind engages the world lovingly and creatively (*libido*), or hatefully and destructively (*death-drive*).[1].Particularly in the very early years of childhood, drive cathects a person's own parents through a progressive development in *autoerotic, narcissistic, oral, anal, phallic,* and *Oedipal* stages.[2] Because of its incestuous nature, abhorrent to the moral mind of later childhood and adulthood, much of this early experience is completely forgotten or *repressed.* Normally, a person's forgotten ancient past, which has shaped adult drive, smoothly coordinates with later mental functioning. However, if a real or imagined trauma has occurred during early childhood, drive does not develop normally but is *fixated* and *de-fused* (so that "the past haunts the present"). Because of fixation, the memories which had been repressed are constantly returning as symptoms, which are *compromise-formations* between the will of the repressed and the repressive, or of the id, ego, and superego, associatively linked to the pathogenic memories in their specific features, and resulting in hysteria (repressed feelings converted into physical symptoms), obsessional thoughts and ritualistic compulsions, phobias and fetishes. Because of de-fusion, death-drive phenomena such as excessive hatred, self-reproach, and self-destructiveness, are pronounced.

Relevant for our purposes, psychodynamic theory clarified the nature of the psychic traumas that play such an important role in mental pathogenesis—the so-called *danger situations.*[3] These potential catastrophes have a special power to scar the ego during its early development, and cause pain and distress when encountered in later life, particularly in those individuals in whom they reactivate unconscious memories of an earlier trauma. They include loss of the *object* (i.e., parent figure on whom one depends), loss of the object's love, castration, and loss of the superego's (or moral agency's) love. Familiarity with the danger situations brings a wealth of wisdom to psychiatric practice, especially in a potentially traumatizing milieu like the emergency room (and hospital to which it is attached) where many of these situations can be re-enacted, at least in the patient's unconscious mind.

The unfortunate patient of our case presented with vengeful hatred toward the doctors who had removed his testicle, thereby exposing him to the classic danger situation of castration. The psychodynamic method of listening considers the patient's injury and its impact in the here-and-now, while also keeping in mind that historical traumas may have been unconsciously reactivated by the current injury, reinforcing its emotional effects. Therefore, from a psychodynamic perspective, the traumatic event itself condenses current events with historical trauma and their emotional effects. The resulting psychiatric symptoms are considered *multi-determined,* that is, caused not only by the present trauma, but by one or more historical traumas. In our case, the details of the patient's early life were completely unknown, but it is possible that his extreme mental reaction to the orchidectomy signaled an awakening of unconscious memories of related early traumas, perhaps providing a clue that he had been raised in a castrating environment during his Oedipal phase (approximately age 3–6), when his drive to engage with the world manifesting as natural curiosity in its direct sexual or *sublimated* (i.e., nonsexual or cultural) forms was interfered with by parental abuse or *sadism,* or insufficient love and protection. This potentially traumatic developmental milieu, which he did not explicitly describe, but which we are *reconstructing* from some of the details of his clinical presentation, may account for his inadequate development and chronic low functioning. Although the well-intentioned surgeons were hardly to blame for this man's problems, his vengeful hatred, originally directed toward the parents who had abused or neglected (i.e., "castrated") him, was *projected* outward and *displaced* onto them. It is a psychological mechanism that is prone to occur, for as we know from psychodynamic theory, the libidinal position is relatively fixed while its objects are changeable. It would be remiss here to not mention the possibility that his incurring the injury in the first place, or his neglect to get the proper care for it, could be driven by the *repetition compulsion*, the inexorable drive to repeat traumatic scenarios in the quest to reverse roles and achieve mastery (i.e., become the aggressor).

Awareness of the psychodynamic aspects of this case are less relevant to some components of the clinical encounter, such as the diagnostic, safety, and capacity evaluations, but would inform the clinician's attitude toward the patient and, it is hoped, enhance his empathy and tact.[4] With regard to empathy, the psychodynamic method allows for a more comprehensive understanding of the patient because it focuses attention not just on the here-and-now but the echoing aftereffects of early-life trauma by also listening with a historically conscious ear. With regard to tact, the psychodynamically informed clinician realizes that they are another authority figure who could potentially be *internalized* as a superego figure or *parental imago*, thus potentially modifying the patient's most important relationship of all, which is his relationship toward himself. Using a loose definition, the attachment and feelings the patient develops toward the clinician based on prior traumas and experiences can be termed *transference*. Understanding that this process is unconscious for the patient can be freeing for the clinician in that it allows them to avoid feeling that attacks are personal in nature. The tactful clinician would be especially careful not to re-traumatize the patient, by trying not to sadistically attack him even in a subtle away, even if provoked, or to abandon his needs, or to deal with him disrespectfully.[5] Even in the full knowledge that early traumas, as this man is speculated to have suffered, are particularly resistant to treatment, the psychiatrist always must endeavor to be internalized as a good object (not through special heroic acts, but through simple care, respect, and *neutrality*) and not to be internalized as a bad object. For those excited by the clinical task, it is gratifying to realize that every clinical encounter in the emergency room could be an opportunity for psychodynamic healing.

While this first case served as an introduction to psychodynamic principles, the subsequent two will show more challenging, but common, clinical scenarios that placed greater emotional demands on the clinician and where the conceptual lens afforded by psychodynamic theory was particularly needed.

CASE 2: METABOLIZING NEGATIVE COUNTERTRANSFERENCE

A 24-year-old Korean-born adoptee student with no formal psychiatric history was brought into the emergency room by ambulance after a reported suicide attempt. Clinical history revealed that her boyfriend had broken up with her, and she was texting a school friend about how she was cutting herself and having suicidal thoughts. On mental status examination, she was calm, cooperative, sad and tearful. Fresh very superficial lacerations were visible on her tattooed arms. She admitted that she had been having suicidal thoughts earlier that night, but denied current suicidal thoughts, was willing to start an antidepressant for dysthymia which underlay the adjustment reaction she was presenting with, and seemed appreciative of the opportunity to receive follow-up care in the hospital's crisis clinic. The clinician was aware of having a countertransference response of the "heroic rescuer," of having forged a connection, which cut through the fatigue, warmed his heart, and even made him feel glad to be busily working on a holiday weekend at 3:30 A.M.

Treatment Issues

Not wanting to minimize the patient's suicide risk, the clinician contacted the school friend with the patient's permission. The friend said that the patient had had a series of recent break-ups with this boyfriend, and it was not the first time she had mentioned suicide, which had alarmed the friend greatly and made her unsure what to do—she certainly had thought of calling an ambulance in the past. She felt the patient was a suicide risk and urged the clinician to not discharge her. After this phone call, the clinician was now feeling like it would probably be the prudent thing and legally justifiable to hospitalize the patient voluntarily or involuntarily. As he was reporting this change of plan to the patient, her sad calmness transformed into rage. She began attacking the clinician, yelling "Let me out of here— I want to go home!," and adding for good measure, "You're probably shitty at what you do, because I know all the good psychiatrists are in private practice." She suddenly got up from her chair, and exited the room, slamming the door behind her. She could still be heard yelling at the top of her lungs. Feeling angry, humiliated, and even betrayed, the clinician asked the nurse to prepare sedating medications.

Psychodynamic Aspects of the Case

An influential school within psychodynamic theory is *object relations* which particularly shed light on the mental structures and mechanisms underlying severe e-motional disturbance, intersubjective dynamics in the physician-patient relationship, and the clinical uses of countertransference.

As it is instructive to see how the mental structure of more disturbed patients differs from that of healthier, neurotic-level patients, let us first consider the latter. In normal or neurotic individuals, at the end of the Oedipal period, the infantile sexual bonds with the parent are ruptured.[6] As a consequence of this watershed psychic event, which marks the end of early childhood, the parent (i.e., the former love object) is taken into the child's own ego and becomes a psychic object. Another name for the parental psychic object is the *superego*. In psychologically healthy individuals who had a protective, loving bond with a parent figure during early childhood, the ego-superego is the nucleus of the psyche.

In individuals who lacked that bond, there was no *object permanence*, and/or *object constancy*, and this nucleus never formed. Instead, these unfortunate so-called *borderline* individuals are postulated to have a poorly structuralized psyche composed of multiple positively and negatively valenced self-object dyads bound together by primitive and intense affects (also referred to as *superego precursors*), the precipitates of its abortive attempts at loving and being loved.[7]

The usual stress response of the borderline patient's psyche is *splitting*. Not only are the good dyads split off from the bad dyads (so that the borderline patient experiences him- or herself and others as all-good or all-bad), but under the least stress, splitting within dyads also occurs, and consequently a bad or good self- or object-representation is projected onto others.

In these cases, subject-object indeterminacy characterizes the clinical dyad. Under the stress of her current situation and determined by her needs, the patient of our case unconsciously projected a heroically loving object-representation onto the clinician who was immediately drawn in. Building on the prior definition of transference, countertransference can be understood as the feelings that the clinician experiences toward the patient, based on both the patient's behavior and projections and the clinician's own background and development. The alien affect states he felt were a countertransference cue that his psyche had been invaded, warping his responses by the process of *projective identification*.

When she got frustrating news, this patient's mood, demeanor, and attitude rapidly changed. Consistent with a poorly consolidated superego, she displayed intense and primitive emotions including feelings of abandonment and betrayal, and a lack of self-regulation, moral constraint, and empathy (recall her "you're a shitty psychiatrist!" barb).

Elicited by her attacks, the usually sober-minded physician now felt projected onto him a vengeful cruel object-representation. Here is where the critical intervention occurred: as he was telling the nurse to draw up the injection, he became aware of his own heightened emotions—anger, vengefulness, and sadism—toward the patient, telltale signs of the patient's invading object-representation. By reflecting on his own emotions, he was able to *metabolize* these invasive affects and attitudes. Back in an emotionally neutral state, and now wishing to calmly care for and regulate the patient as a *good-enough* parent, mature superego or adequately functioning clinician should do, he realized it might be possible to verbally "talk her down" instead of exposing her to potential re-traumatization by a restraint procedure. He also became aware that other patients, some fearfully, others opportunistically, had tuned in to see whether control or dyscontrol would prevail in the mind of the clinician and on the milieu. The clinician explained the need for the patient to stay quiet and in control to protect her, other patients', and staff safety with the consequence of being medicated if she could not do so, but she refused to look at or acknowledge him, mutely holding the sheet over her face. Upon returning to the nursing station, he heard her banging her fist on the plastic window of the observation bay and screaming, and in the end the patient required sedation for her own safety.

In summary, particularly with borderline patients, the psychiatric clinician must be aware of and actively manage his or her countertransference to avoid cruel or super-heroic projective identification responses, and instead be the caring, regulating object these unfortunate patients never experienced during development or could never internalize. While one isolated clinical experience will probably not be curative, it can prevent further harm.

CASE 3: COUNTERTRANSFERENCE AS A SOURCE OF ERROR

A 28-year-old white man was brought in by ambulance to a busy emergency room on a Saturday evening. In a carefully controlled but imperious manner, he pleaded with the nurses to have the doctor evaluate him as soon as possible. The nurse poked her head into the doctor's area to report with a smirk that "Mr. X is asking to be seen, he said he needs to catch a flight!" The doctor actually did choose to see him out of turn, perhaps with some such rationale as: other patients could wait, and this apparently impatient patient might "escalate." At a less conscious level, he might have been aware that this patient, by trying to break the routine, was challenging his authority, which piqued his competitiveness and aggression: he was going to show him who was boss!

Mental status exam revealed a tired-appearing young blond-haired man in an Oxford shirt and slacks. Throughout the interview, the clinician had the sense that the patient was "going through the motions" to talk his way out of an undesirable situation. The patient opened the interview by saying "This is all a mistake!" First of all, he didn't need to be here because he already had a psychiatrist who treated him for ADHD and prescribed Adderall. Second, it was his girlfriend's mother who had been meddling via text message as he and his girlfriend were breaking up, and who had called 911. Admittedly, it had been a tumultuous few days. One of his own family members was severely ill. He had been with his girlfriend in the Midwest visiting that family member. Circumstances had him reflecting on his own life choices, and he was speaking with his girlfriend about his dissatisfaction with his high-paying, prestigious, but back-breaking "partner-track" position at a famous financial institution, and how he was considering transitioning careers. The girlfriend was alarmed and protesting, it escalated into a break-up fight, and he ended up flying back without her.

Then there was the text messaging, with the girlfriend's mother getting involved—the details of it all he said he could not recall or were not worth recalling, but he vehemently denied making suicidal or homicidal threats, or saying anything "psychotic." Back in his apartment, he drank a couple beers and then went for a jog. Soon after he returned, the police were knocking at his door. He decided to hide under his bed. The police entered with guns drawn, and then called an ambulance to bring him to the hospital. He thought it was all "ludicrous." One further detail: his employer was sending him to Europe on a "$14,000" flight early the next morning and it was imperative that he be discharged.

Treatment Issues

The clinician noticed that the patient was focused on the goal of being discharged, and being evasive and intentionally withholding important details, as his clinical narrative had plenty of obvious holes. What had he said that prompted the girlfriend's mother to call 911? Why did he hide under the bed when the police arrived? What did he say to police that prompted them to call an ambulance? Although the patient was "holding it together" pretty well in the emergency room, either primary or secondary mania (perhaps caused by substance use) certainly were plausible diagnostic considerations. Getting an outside perspective, preferably from the girlfriend's mother and perhaps the patient's psychiatrist, was imperative. While recognizing the need to fill in this information, the clinician—who, you will recall, had begun the clinical encounter with the unconscious desire to assert his authority over a demanding and disruptive patient—would also have admitted that he had already decided to discharge this patient and was not inclined to spend much more time investigating the case. The manner in which clinical contact changed the clinician's attitude leading to a hasty decision was the interesting and consequential part of the countertransference.

The patient reluctantly provided a phone number apparently from memory which he said was the girlfriend's (he said did not know the girlfriend's mother's number). The clinician called it and it went to a generic voicemail recording (was the number even the girlfriend's?). He left a message, but, before hearing back, he decided to discharge the patient, believing he did not meet "involuntary retention criteria." He felt a sense of relief in informing the patient, who had been calmly but insistently hovering just outside the doctor's area, of this desired outcome. A day later, the patient was brought back by ambulance to the psychiatric emergency room. At that time the full story was revealed: he had been drinking, using cocaine, and sending threatening text messages to the girlfriend and her mother, who had again called 911.

Psychodynamic Aspects of the Case

In this case, a *countertransference blind-spot* perturbed the clinician's normal clinical functioning. Like all symptoms (this one occurring in the clinician instead of the patient) according to the psychodynamic style of thinking, this blind-spot was *multi-determined*. It resulted from the unaware clinician falling under the sway of strong countertransference affects that rendered the patient both repellent and seductive, but also—and this is the important distinction from the previous case example—as healthier than he appeared and needing nothing from the clinician.

The psychodynamic theory of *narcissism* will help us understand these countertransference affects. Narcissism refers to the idea that at the dawn of psychic time, the not yet fully individuated infant experiences himself in a blissful state of perfection in fusion with the parents' projected wishes.[8] A major psychic trauma occurs during that inevitable first moment of parental disapproval or criticism that shatters the child's perfect view of himself and makes the parent a fully separate and threatening figure. This trauma is so massive that it leads to a splitting of the ego, into an ego and new psychic structure called the *ego ideal*. In the normal case, much of a person's self-love now flows onto the internalized ideal standards, or ego ideal, and relatively less onto the imperfect ego, which in fact is tragically doomed to never quite live up to its ideal. In abnormal cases, the realities of the ego's imperfection are too much to bear: under stress, or in response to further traumatic slights that again reinforce the sense of the ego's weakness, there is a multi-part defensive maneuver: repression of the feeling of weakness, and a *psychic regression* (or illusionistic wish-fulfillment) whereby the self is again experienced in a state of *fusion* with the ideal object and ego-ideal (psychic residues of the perfectly-loving parent).[9] In addition, projective defenses are put into play that externalize the ego's weaknesses, and they are instead perceived in others. As a consequence of all this, the state of perfection is partially recovered but at the price of a grandiose view of oneself and an arrogantly dismissive view of others.

How did the patient's narcissistic pathology interfere with the clinician's intention to deliver appropriate care?

As the theory describes, the purely narcissistic individual uses a primitive defensive maneuver to avoid needing anything from others (who, according to the theory, can only hurt and devalue). Somewhat paradoxically, this often includes refusing, or having only limited acceptance of, the patient role. Consequently, psychodynamic wisdom recognizes *narcissistic inaccessibility* as one of the emotional attitudes that makes patients essentially untreatable as it renders them unreceptive to the influence of a healing "object" (instead, they re-invest all their libido in themselves).[10] Had he been more aware of his countertransference, the clinician would have realized that the patient's narcissistic inaccessibility elicited feelings of distance and clinical futility.

The regression and fusion of the narcissist with his own ego ideal can also stir up other countertransference affects. Since the clinical manifestation of this process is sickness illusionistically masquerading as vigor and health, the narcissistic patient can have taboo-like and enchanting powers. Unconsciously guided by *reaction-formation*, the narcissistic patient is often able to find a successful adaptation to the working world and its hierarchies, where she/he can obtain and exercise power (recall that this patient had a "partner-track" position at a famous financial firm). Our patient's markers of status and success which he flaunted as a kind of ego armor, and his highly restrained grandiosity and contempt, were liable to elicit countertransference attitudes of over-identification, admiration, and deferential fear in the clinician. If the clinician's own character is vulnerable—which is not unlikely, for some degree of narcissism is probably ubiquitous, as narcissistic trauma is probably a universal stage in psycho-ontogenesis—a patient like this can even trigger a narcissistic reaction, setting off an unconscious wish in the clinician to fuse with the patient as with an (external, i.e., projected) ideal ego.[11]

Finally, the patient's externalizing defenses (somewhat muted toward the clinician in this case, because the patient, being trapped in the ED, was careful not to insult the person who had power over his fate) made the clinician feel *devaluated*, eliciting anger and aversion.

Whereas the previous case showed how countertransference when properly metabolized is a potent, even a necessary, psychiatric tool, this case shows how unmetabolized countertransference disrupts care. Fueled by a mix of unprocessed affects such as distance, futility and, aversion which made him dislike the narcissistic patient; as well as over-identification, admiration and deferential fear, which made him under-pathologize and want to appease the patient; the clinician lapsed into an *enactment* by prematurely discharging him. Because the patient's intolerable behavior resulted in him being brought back to the emergency room the next day, the consequences of this clinical error were the mild one of professional embarrassment for the clinician, but they could have been dangerous or even fatal for the patient and/or others.

Generally speaking, narcissistic patients can be a particularly challenging clinical population in the emergency room because their defensive structure makes them likely to resist the patient role and display traits of apparent health, which may deflect attention away from the co-existing presence of sometimes very severe psychiatric illness. Because of the countertransferences these patients give rise to, and the rage they may feel if they don't get their way (as this patient could very well have unleashed if the clinician had retained him), special efforts at countertransference awareness, emotional tolerance and clinical rigor are often required.

DISCUSSION

In the preceding pages, libido, object relations, and narcissism components of psychodynamic theory were used to understand the clinical dynamics of three cases in the psychiatric emergency room. Our particular focus on countertransference confirms the truth of the adage that opened this chapter: even in the emergency room, while face to face with patients, the clinician often must do or say nothing while actively reflecting upon countertransference affects—allowing him or her to see and think more deeply, make unimpeded decisions, and relate to patients with greater empathy and tact. Indeed, from the material in this chapter, it becomes evident that the emergency room places particular demands on the psychodynamic skill of the clinician. Where there is a high volume of unknown and unpredictable patients; untreated illness often accompanied by intense affects and potentially dangerous behaviors; and a primary clinical task of sorting out who is severely ill from who is not, the clinician's clearest possible perception of self and others is paramount. Such clarity is required both for the optimal triage and initial management of individual patients, and for assuring all patients and staff that a competent and trustworthy authority governs the milieu.

Key Clinical Points

- Understanding normal development and the impact on personality function and structure that disrupted development can cause can be helpful for the ED clinician encountering patients in crisis.
- Monitoring and metabolizing countertransferential reactions can increase empathy as well as decrease impulsive and unconscious acting out in the clinical relationship.
- Blind spots in clinician judgment can occur in reaction to narcissistic or borderline patients. Understanding and anticipating adverse reactions can help clinicians maintain a therapeutic and safe frame for evaluation and treatment.

REFERENCES

1. Freud S, Strachey J (trans.). *New introductory lectures on psychoanalysis*. New York, NY: Norton; 1965.
2. Freud S, Strachey J (trans.). *Three essays on the theory of sexuality*. New York, NY: Basic Books; 1975.
3. Freud S. *Inhibitions, symptoms and anxiety*. New York, NY: Norton; 1977.
4. Schafer R. *The analytic attitude*. London: Karnac Books; 1983.
5. Strachey J. The nature of the therapeutic action of psycho-analysis. *The journal of psychotherapy practice and research* 1999; 8(1):66–82.
6. Freud S, Strachey J (trans.). The Dissolution of the Oedipus Complex. *The standard edition of the complete psychological works of Sigmund Freud, Volume XIX (1923–1925)*. London: Hogarth Press, 1961.

7. Caligor E, Kernberg OF, Clarkin JF. *Handbook of dynamic psychotherapy for higher level personality pathology.* Arlington, VA: American Psychiatric Publishing; 2007.

8. Freud S, Strachey J (trans.). On Narcissism: An Introduction. *The standard edition of the complete psychological works of Sigmund Freud, Volume XIV (1914–16).* London: Hogarth Press, 1957.

9. Kernberg OF. Factors in the psychoanalytic treatment of narcissistic personalities. *Journal of the American Psychoanalytic Association* 1970; 18:51–85.

10. Freud S. The Economic Problem of Masochism. *The standard edition of the complete psychological works of Sigmund Freud, Volume XIX (1923–1925).* London: Hogarth Press, 1961.

11. Groves JE, Dunderdale BA, Stern TA. Celebrity patients, VIPs, and potentates. *Primary care companion to the journal of clinical psychiatry* 2002; 4(6):215–223.

16

Use of Interpreters in Emergency Psychiatric Evaluation

BIPIN SUBEDI AND KATHERINE MALOY ■

CASE HISTORY: THE AGITATED PATIENT WHO DOES NOT SPEAK ENGLISH

Mr. B, a 30-year-old Bengali man, was brought to the emergency room by local police after he was found agitated in front of a local store. Accompanying documents indicate that the storeowner called 911 because Mr. B was yelling about "wanting money" and refused to leave the premises. Police reported that the patient was banging on the windows of the storefront, "harassing" customers, and used the word "die."

Upon presentation to the hospital Mr. B was able to communicate in English on a basic level. He said he was "very sad" because he was far away from his family and was "worry about money." He said he was previously selling "shirt" on the street and was "mad" that the storeowner had not paid him despite two weeks of work. Any attempts to obtain additional information about recent events resulted in perseveration about the money he was owed and the resulting "stress." He denied any violent thoughts but quickly returned to the earlier themes anytime he was asked about his recent agitation. He said he was "good, good" when asked about sleep, appetite, and concentration. He said, "No die" when asked about suicide and said, "Yes" when asked if he was "hearing voices."

Mr. B was noted to be deferential to the treatment team but pleaded for release and "help." He stated that he was given medication for "problem sleeping" in Bangladesh, but was unable to provide additional details. He said, "No, no" when asked if he ever tried to harm himself, but quickly shifted into discussing how he was struggling to make ends meet in America. He responded similarly when attempts were made to assess past mania and psychosis. He said he had been "sad" when his father died in Bangladesh but otherwise was dismissive when the team inquired about any history of depression. Mr. B reported that he completed the equivalent of college and worked for his family's business for several years before coming to the United States for a "better life." He said he lived in an apartment with another Bengali man but did not have his roommate's phone number.

Collateral Contact: The storeowner was called for collateral information. He said Mr. B has been selling various items on a local street corner for several months. He said that he occasionally hires the patient to clean the store but had noticed recently that he seemed distracted, easily angered and was taking to himself. He said Mr. B was "acting crazy" on the morning of presentation and accused the storeowner of withholding payment although he had been paid, as usual, after the completion of his shift the prior evening. He was not able to provide the names or phone number of additional contacts.

Mental Status Exam: On examination Mr. B was slightly disheveled but otherwise well groomed and cooperative. He had fair eye contact that became intense when describing his frustration with the storeowner. He also shifted in his seat and waved his arms around during these times. His speech was pressured and loud. His thought process seemed overly inclusive, loose and perseverative.

Mr. B repeatedly refused to use an interpreter service saying that his "English good," and asked to leave if the team could not help him recover the money that was owed to him. Initial attempts to educate him on the potential benefits of interpreter services were unsuccessful. Finally, the evaluating clinician repeated multiple times that the patient could not be released until he agreed to speak with the phone interpreter, and he eventually complied.

Interview with Interpreter: Using the phone interpreter the team discovered that Mr. B came to America one year ago to live with his uncle because he believed his parents were sabotaging his efforts to obtain employment in his native country. He left this apartment several months earlier after he started "noticing" that his uncle was also interfering with his attempts to find a job. He initially slept on the streets but has been staying in a shelter in the basement of a local mosque over the last month. He said that he had been "very worried" that the mosque leadership was trying to harm him and, the day prior, noticed a strange mark on a ten-dollar bill that he was given by the storeowner. He said that he "knows" that the money is "fake" and returned to the store that day to demand proper payment. Mr. B could not offer a clear explanation of why he was given a counterfeit bill, saying only, "Like my family."

The interpreter noted that the patient repeatedly made reference to his parents being "devils," which is an odd term to use given his cultural and religious background. She often had to ask the same question multiple times to keep the Mr. B on topic and noted that at times he "didn't make any sense." She clarified that the patient assumed the physicians were assessing his hearing when they asked about auditory hallucinations, and Mr. B denied hearing any sounds or noises when alone. He said he had not been sleeping regularly over concerns that he would be attacked at night, leading him to be tired and "confused" at times during the day. He said he was feeling depressed because of recent events but denied any plan to harm himself. Despite all this, he was adamant that the storeowner needed to pay him and wanted to be released so he could get "real money" from him.

Disposition: Mr. B recognized that his life had been increasingly stressful recently and recalled that medication had been helpful in treating his insomnia in the past. He admitted that he did not feel like "himself," and identified target symptoms of anxiety and irritability. He indicated that he had originally assumed that the doctors worked for the authorities but now felt that they could be helpful in making him feel better. Mr. B eventually agreed to sign into the hospital voluntarily for treatment after further clarification of the admission process.

CASE 2: THE DEAF PATIENT

A 32-year-old white woman with unknown prior psychiatric history presents to the emergency department accompanied by a friend. She appears agitated and has difficulty standing still. She does not speak, but her friend informs the nurse that they are both deaf, and that her friend will require an American Sign Language (ASL) interpreter. The friend brought the patient for increasingly bizarre behavior over the past week and notes she might have a history of psychiatric treatment, but she is not sure. They both work at a school for deaf children.

While waiting for the interpreter, the patient is noted to be signing rapidly to her friend who is trying to keep her calm. As it is after regular business hours, the triage nurse uses a video relay service to provide ASL interpretation via a video terminal. An interpreter is accessed quickly, however, the interpreter quickly notes that she is having difficulty seeing the patient's extremely rapid movements due to some slight video lag, and the patient becomes frustrated and storms out of the room.

Collateral Contact: While waiting for an in-person interpreter, some history is taken from the patient's friend, who is able to lip-read and speak. She has known the patient for two years as a co-worker and friend. She notes the patient finished college and works as a teacher of deaf children, she is a reliable employee. She has mentioned seeing a therapist, but the friend does not know for what. The friend does not think she uses drugs, and they have been out socially together where the patient has appeared to drink very little. Then the triage nurse attempts to interview the patient through writing, but the patient also quickly becomes frustrated.

Interview with Interpreter: After the in-person interpreter arrives, the patient is visibly relieved, and the nurse, doctor and social worker all meet together with the patient to maximize the interpreter's time. The patient is still difficult to understand, with ideas and phrases coming very rapidly and in a disorganized manner. She gets up and paces several times and seems to believe the interpreter knows what she is thinking and is simply withholding information to be difficult. The team is able to piece together that she has not slept in a week, that she believes she has been given a special and divine purpose, and that she can't stop her thoughts. She did not want to come today to the hospital because she has to heal people and save the planet as she has been directed. She has continued teaching this week but notes that the staff at the school don't understand her and she is now very frustrated with all of them for not realizing how important she is and is going to quit her job and move away somewhere. She is able to state that she doesn't have any medical problems and doesn't use any drugs or alcohol. She does allude to a prior incident in college where she did not sleep more than a few hours a night for several weeks and suddenly became extremely productive and irritable. The episode subsided on its own, and she denies ever being hospitalized.

Disposition: The psychiatrist is sufficiently convinced that the patient is most likely experiencing an acute manic episode. She takes the opportunity of having the interpreter present to discuss the possibility of this diagnosis with the patient and advise her that she may need to be hospitalized briefly for stabilization. The patient is reluctant to be hospitalized, but does agree that she feels increasingly afraid and uncomfortable with how she cannot slow down her thinking.

All laboratory studies are normal, toxicology is negative, and the patient—with reassurance from her friend—is eventually admitted voluntarily to the hospital for stabilization.

DISCUSSION

Studies have shown that non-English speaking patients are more likely to receive sub-optimal medical care.[1] Medical evaluations for these clients can be frustrating for both the patient and clinician. The patient may feel confused about the purpose of questioning, especially if they have underlying psychiatric symptoms that impair communication. Clinicians, who are often juggling multiple patients in a busy ED, may be inclined to accept basic English to avoid the time associated with obtaining information via interpreter services. Patients may also avoid requesting an interpreter due to fear of stigmatization, or wish to expedite the evaluation.

However, diagnostic assessment and treatment planning requires a thorough examination and collection of accurate data. The first part of the clinical encounter should be geared toward building rapport and determining the level of English proficiency necessary for proper communication. This includes asking the non-native English speaker if they prefer to use interpreter services. If the clinician determines that interpreter services are needed, then they should be used. If the patient is resistant to this, the focus should be to encourage them to accept this intervention.

Use of sign language interpretation is similar to use of any other medical language interpreter, in that it requires rapport with the patient, a skilled interpreter who has knowledge of medical issues, and adds a layer of complexity to the evaluation. It is also important to remember that just as a group of people who speak the same language may have vastly different cultural backgrounds, deaf and hard-of-hearing individuals are a diverse group. Given the multiplicity of causes of deafness, varying ages at which deafness occurs and differences in education, the emergency department provider may have to troubleshoot their communication strategy to fit the patient's abilities. A 90- year-old who has age-related hearing loss and a poorly functioning hearing aid is obviously different from this patient, who was deaf from birth. However, this patient—as evidenced by her completing college and working full time—is also different from a patient who may also have intellectual disabilities from the illness that led to their deafness, or who may also have vision impairment. Even deaf individuals with relatively similar intellectual abilities may have had vastly different educational backgrounds. In this case, the patient had minimal lip-reading and no speech and what lip-reading skill she had was drastically impaired by her acute manic symptoms and resulting irritability. Her friend, also congenitally deaf, had been educated in a setting where she learned both ASL and some speech, and thus served as a very helpful escort. ASL is a unique language that has its own grammar. It is not a word-for-word translation of English, which makes learning both spoken and written English and ASL difficult, particularly if the individual is not educated in both from early childhood. Deaf individuals who can write and read in English as well as sign fluently are essentially bilingual. Thus it is possible, depending on educational background, for someone to sign fluently but not be able to use written English as an adequate method of communication. Finally, deaf individuals from other counties may have different sign languages that make interpretation even more challenging.

Similarly, while it is helpful to have some basic understanding of the different cultural backgrounds of non-English speaking patients in the environment in which a clinician works, it is also important to anticipate diversity within a language or culture. Patients who are Spanish speaking, for example, can have vastly different backgrounds and countries of origin, and patients from the same country of origin may have very different socioeconomic or religious backgrounds.

Interpreter services can helpful in obtaining historical narratives in addition to concrete symptoms. Assessing psychotic symptoms can be particularly challenging in non-English speaking patients.[2] Experienced interpreters may be able to offer opinions with regards to thought form was well as cultural and religious norms. Difficulty communicating in English may present as agitation, and it is important to distinguish this from underlying mood or psychotic symptoms. Similarly, awkward phrasing in English can be lost in translation and lead to additional confusion.

In person, professionally trained interpreters should be used when possible. However, this service is often not always available for low-frequency languages, and in these cases phone services are an acceptable substitute. Care should be taken in evaluating an agitated or violent patient when using an object such as a phone. Video relay technology has made sign language interpretation more accessible, but it also has limitations, particularly if patients are also visually impaired, and it relies on an internet connection that may vary as to its quality. In the case discussed, the patient was signing too rapidly for the video interpreter to follow given the limits of the video streaming service.

The interpreter can be viewed as an extension of the person being evaluated. Both the interpreter and patient should sit together, across from and facing the clinician. The person interviewing should speak directly to the patient to maximize use of eye contact, gestures, and other forms of non-verbal communication. This will also help further the patient-clinician relationship and build rapport. Interpreters should provide word-for-word translation; it important to pause for the interpreter and to break up longer statements or explanations into smaller fragments in order to minimize the chances of important information or ideas being lost. Attempts should be made to avoid the use of medical terminology as equivalent words or ideas may not exist in other languages. For example, asking, "Have you been feeling worried or stressed about anything lately?" may be more helpful then inquiring about "anxiety." Similarly, asking, "Do you ever hear any noises or sounds that others cannot?" or, "do you ever hear people talking when you are in a room alone?" are ways to probe for auditory hallucinations.

Clinicians should educate themselves on the stressors experienced by ethnic groups in their local area. Some minorities may be more likely to be undocumented and others may tend to have significant debts related to paying for immigration-related services. Both of these issues can lead to economic pressure that necessitates working long hours or traveling extended distances for employment, as well as time away from family and friends. Awareness of the political, cultural and economic climate of immigrant populations, particularly refugees, can help the clinician build rapport and appreciate psychosocial stressors.[3] Knowing the religion of a certain ethic group may help identify local supports at areas of worship. Understanding the structure of patient's living situation can be useful in identifying additional stressors as well as supports. Patients without family in the United States may be living with other members of their community in shared housing for financial reasons. In the first case, the interpreter was also helpful in providing cultural context that the patient's ideas were not in fact congruent with his religious beliefs.

Working with deaf patients can also have particular cultural challenges. While some deaf individuals function within a mostly hearing world, others are ensconced in a deaf culture where most of their friends, colleagues and family members are also deaf, or also sign. This patient worked in a school for deaf children, and thus spent most of her life around people who sign. Many outpatient settings are not equipped to provide treatment to deaf individuals, thus further complicating disposition and referral. A 1995 study showed that while a majority of physicians understood that ASL interpretation was the most appropriate method of communicating with deaf patients, only 22% used it regularly in their practice.[4] A 2004 study interviewing deaf patients about their experiences in health care settings did not show much improvement.[5] Deaf patients already face significant hurdles in obtaining mental health care[6] and the emergency psychiatric setting can be even more challenging, given that there is usually an ongoing crisis that precipitated the visit.

Hospitalization in a setting where no one else signs or speaks the patient's native language, and where the only communication available a once-daily meeting with an interpreter can be alienating and frightening. In addition, coordinating social supports can be more challenging when there are communication barriers. One strategy if in-person interpretation is available is to meet with the patient as a team when the interpreter is present, to maximize the interpreter's time, and to make sure everyone is aware of the patient's concerns.

Interpreters can provide psychoeducation and clarification for clients who may be confused about the treatment and evaluation processes in the United States. This is especially true for patients coming from countries where there are limited resources or reasons to distrust authority figures. In general, it is important to be sensitive to concerns regarding privacy and potential embarrassment that may come with speaking about emotional or psychiatric issues. Spending time normalizing emotional responses and acknowledging challenging experiences can be helpful in creating a safe space for open discussion.

Key Clinical Points

- Language and culture are important factors in psychiatric evaluation. While interpretation adds a layer of complexity to the evaluation, it is also essential to obtaining clear clinical picture.
- Patients who do not speak English or who are deaf or hard of hearing may experience healthcare settings as alienating and frightening. Extra care should be taken in making sure the patient is understood and their needs appreciate.
- Language interpretation should be readily accessible and easy to access, particularly in the ED setting.

REFERENCES

1. Ramirez D, Engel K, Tang T. language interpreter utilization in the emergency department setting: a clinical review. *Journal of Health Care for the Poor and Underserved* 2008; 19:352–362.
2. Bauer A, Margarita A. The impact of patient language proficiency and interpreter service use on the quality of psychiatric care: A systematic review. *Psychiatric Services* 2010; 61:765–773.
3. Crosby S. Primary care management of non–English-speaking refugees who have experienced trauma: A clinical review. *Journal of the American Medical Association* 2013; 310:519–528.
4. Ebert D, Heckerling, P. Communication with deaf patients: knowledge, belief and practices of physicians. *Journal of the American Medical Association.* 1995; 273(3):227–229. doi:10.1001/jama.1995.03520270061032
5. Lezzoni L, O'Day B, Killeen M, et al. Communicating about healthcare: Observations from persons who are deaf or hard of hearing. *Annals of Internal Medicine* 2004; 140(5):356–362. doi:10.7326/0003-4819-140-5-200403020-
6. Steinberg AG, Sullivan VJ, Loew RC. Cultural and linguistic barriers to mental health services: A consumer perspective. *American Journal of Psychiatry* 1998 Jul; 155(7):982–984.

17

Evaluating and Treating
the Homeless Patient

KATHERINE MALOY ∎

CASE 1: THE NEW ARRIVAL

History of Present Illness: A 23-year-old white man with a history of anxiety and ADHD walks in to the emergency department (ED) requesting medication refills. He reports to the triage nurse that he moved across the country to stay with a friend he primarily had interacted with for the last few years online. When he arrived, the friend was able to house him only for a short time. The apartment was crowded with other people and drug use was rampant. The patient did not end up getting the job he had hoped for, and has been intermittently using alcohol and marijuana. He has now run out of the medications (sertraline, alprazolam and amphetamine/dextroamphetemine) that he states has taken for the last three years. His friend told him that he has to leave the apartment as it is an illegal sublet, and the primary tenant's lease has expired. He has little money, nowhere to stay, and found himself at a homeless drop-in center this afternoon, where they advised him to go to the hospital to get a refill of his medication, as he is starting to feel pretty anxious about his situation. "The people in that homeless shelter . . . they kind of freak me out."

Past Psychiatric History: The patient reports treatment since adolescence for anxiety and ADHD. He has never been hospitalized. He was arrested once for marijuana possession in his home state. He denies a history of violence.

Medical History: No medical problems. No major past hospitalizations.

Social/Developmental: The patient completed high school but dropped out of college in his second year due to poor academic performance leading him to lose his scholarship. He was transiently housed with friends and working odd jobs in his home state. He has intermittent contact with his parents. He had Medicaid coverage in his home state but has not transferred benefits yet.

Laboratory Studies: He has refused to provide a urine drug screen.

Learning Point: Is This Patient Homeless?

This man, despite not meeting usual stereotypes of homeless individuals, has no legal address and no current residence. Most homeless people are transiently homeless, and remain homeless for short periods of time.[1] While he may have a place to stay if he returned to his home state, at least on initial investigation, it seems he has no permanent legal address, and has not had one in some time.

Disposition: The patient was unable or unwilling to provide contact information or even a name of the doctor that had last prescribed his reported medications, and was unwilling to cooperate with laboratory studies or a drug screen, arguing that those procedures were not required in his past treatment. He was ambivalent about remaining in the city, and was interested in hearing about options for travel grants or alternative shelters to the one he had visited. He was offered but refused a follow-up appointment at a free clinic, and elected to return to the drop-in center to see if they would assist him with a bus ticket back to his home state.

CASE 2: THE CHRONICALLY HOMELESS PATIENT

History of Present Illness: A 54-year-old man with a history of schizoaffective disorder, prior state hospitalizations, and multiple arrests for cocaine possession is removed to the hospital from a train station. He also is rumored to have a history of arrest for a sex offense, but this has never been proven. He has multiple similar presentations to the ED, brought by police for behavioral issues in the subway or train stations, or by homeless outreach teams who persuade him to come in to get help. Today he presents having been removed by a homeless outreach team in conjunction with the police, after he was refusing to leave a train station and "aggressively panhandling." He is noted to be disheveled, wearing dirty clothes, smells of alcohol and is mumbling to himself. On interview, he is mostly uncooperative and asks repeatedly to leave. He had stayed at a shelter that is located on the outskirts of the city, but he prefers not to stay there as there are fewer panhandling opportunities, as well as it being heavily populated with men who have recently been in prison. After a long silence, he tells the doctor evaluating him, "There's nothing you can do for me, at least don't make me stay here."

Past Psychiatric History: The patient has multiple prior hospitalizations, as well as several jail terms for low-level drug or "nuisance" offenses such as loitering or sleeping on the train. Thee are vague reports of a history of violence or possible sex offender status, he was in the state hospital over 10 years ago. There is no known history of suicide attempts.

Social History: He has been homeless on the street for several years. History prior to that is unknown.

Medical History: The patient has chronic venous stasis ulcers bilaterally, and has had two brief hospitalizations for cellulitis. He has marginally impaired glucose tolerance, but has never taken medications for diabetes.

Laboratory Studies: Notable for mild normocytic anemia, urine toxicology positive for cocaine and alcohol level of 132.

To Admit or Not to Admit?

While admission criteria vary by state, this case could probably be argued either way under most statutes of involuntary psychiatric retention. The patient presents as psychotic, is known to have a history of psychotic illness, has very poor self-care, and has been aggressive and threatening toward strangers in a public setting. However, he is also acutely intoxicated and once the cocaine and alcohol wear off, he will likely be less immediately dangerous. Despite his long and storied history, he is not known to be frankly violent, more of a public nuisance. One could argue that he has a right to live as he pleases, despite causing discomfort for commuters and having what seems to a poor quality of life. In addition, it seems unlikely that psychiatric hospitalization will ameliorate his behavior, as he has had multiple hospitalizations in the past that have not ended his cycle of homelessness, substance abuse and incarceration.

Disposition: This patient was admitted to an Extended Observation Unit, which allows for up to 72 hours of crisis center observation of patients who are acutely dangerous to themselves or others and, per the legal standard, "may" have a mental illness. He was monitored for alcohol withdrawal and did not require any medications. In the course of 48 hours and though having some disorganization of his speech, he did not display any behavior or symptoms that were acutely dangerous to himself or others once his acute intoxication resolved. Attempts were made to link him directly to a street outreach team; however, the patient refused this direct referral. Within a few weeks, he presented again, this time under arrest for possession of cocaine. He was released to police custody. Several months later, after being sentenced and while serving time in jail, he required acute hospitalization on the forensic psychiatry service for agitated and disorganized behavior that did not seem to be directly drug-related. He was stabilized on decanoate haloperidol but then did not follow up after release from jail.

CASE 3: THE HOMELESS FAMILY

History of Present Illness: A 32-year-old woman with four children living in a family shelter is brought to the ER by ambulance for reported depression and possible suicidal ideation. She is tearful on interview and ashamed of her circumstances. She and her four children sleep in one room. They came to the shelter after being evicted due to nonpayment of rent. She reports that her husband was deported and after that she could not pay rent. She was brought by ambulance today after she began crying uncontrollably in her case workers' office. The case worker asked her if she was having thoughts of hurting herself and she could not stop crying long enough to answer the question. Now she has calmed down, but appears dysphoric and withdrawn. She notes that her children have had to change schools due to the move, and they find the shelter frightening. She denies wanting to hurt herself, and states she would never do anything to put her children in danger, but appears depressed, admitting she is not sleeping and spends all night worrying about what will happen to her. The caseworker who sent her to the hospital is concerned, stating that they have heard her yelling at the children and crying in her room. She does not have anyone to assist in caring for her children if she were admitted to the hospital.

Psychiatric History: She denies having any history of psychiatric illness, suicide attempts, violence or arrests, and denies use of drugs or alcohol

Social History: The patient immigrated several years ago, and is possibly undocumented. Two of her children were born in the United States. She works intermittently.

Laboratory Studies: A urine drug screen was negative. Laboratory studies were normal.

To Admit or Not to Admit?

The patient is obviously in distress and may be underreporting her symptoms due to fear of being admitted or losing her children. There does not seem to be anyone available to corroborate her history of not having a history of suicide attempts or mental illness in the past. She has a several significant acute stressors. However, she seemed genuinely concerned about her children and expressed clearly that she would never do anything to harm herself, she simply does not know what to do and is overwhelmed by her current situation.

Disposition: This patient was not admitted to the hospital, and with her permission, her caseworker at the shelter was contacted to discuss what could be done to provide additional assistance. She was given an appointment for follow-up treatment, which she did not keep. Many months later, one of her children was admitted to the child psychiatric unit for depression, and her depressive symptoms were again noted during family meetings. She expressed guilt over her situation and its effect on her children but was not willing to engage in mental health services for herself. The family was still residing in the shelter system but had begun to be eligible for more long-term housing placement.

DISCUSSION

When most people think of someone as being "homeless," many stereotypes come to mind. The street alcoholic, passed out drunk or someone sleeping under a bridge, are typical examples. In reality, many people are closer to being homeless than we would like to believe, or meet criteria for being homeless when they do not fit the stereotype at all. In New York City, for example, the number of homeless individuals approaches 60,000 people, more than could fit in Madison Square Garden, and the majority of those are families and children.[2]

Clarifying housing status is an important part of determining a treatment plan that is appropriate and therefore more likely to be effective.[3] Patients may not mention they are homeless and may not "look" like they are homeless. Homeless patients face many challenges to treatment. Patients living in shelters, for example, risk having their medications stolen or may lost access to their property periodically if they miss a curfew or lose their bed. Patients who sleep outside have even more limited ability to carry medications with them. Parents in homeless families may fear drawing the attention of child protective services if they are found to have a mental illness, and therefore they underreport their symptoms or may be unwilling to be seen taking medications or attending mental health appointments. Having knowledge of the resources available in the system in which you are practicing can help inform treatment recommendations. Does your patient have to be bused nightly to a distant shelter, and if he misses the bus, does he have nowhere to sleep? Is that what is driving him to present nightly to the ED with vague complaints? Does the patient attend a mandated welfare-to-work program that interferes with attending a scheduled follow-up appointment? Are your homeless patients going to be able to obtain the medications that you prescribe after they leave the hospital? How are they going to transport them? Where are they going to store them? Are there even shelters available in the system where you practice, or are homeless patients predominantly sleeping outside? Have your patients experienced physical or sexual trauma? Do they experience taunts and verbal threats or physical violence as a result of their homelessness? Have they been arrested for "nuisance" crimes such as sleeping in parks after hours or loitering?

Exploring why the patient has become homeless is also important in terms of establishing a diagnosis and clarifying social situation. Many people become homeless due to acute financial stressors or a drastic change in their social situation that is not the result of any psychiatric issue. However, mental illness and substance abuse can significantly contribute to both acute and chronic homelessness. The paranoid patient who flees her residence due to delusions or the alcoholic who loses his job and thus his housing are more explicit examples, but people with personality disorders, for example, may have exhausted their social network, be more vulnerable to loss of employment, or have difficulty successfully navigating the social service system. Victims of domestic violence may become homeless to escape violence and be experiencing trauma-related disorders, or be reluctant to reveal the circumstances due to fear of being exposed or shame about their abuse.[4]

According to a 2011 SAMHSA report, 26.2% of homeless patients in shelters nationally meet criteria for a severe mental illness, and 37.4% met criteria for a substance use disorder.[5] In the second case we see a patient who is closer to the stereotype of chronic homelessness. The patient in the second case is considered *chronically homeless* as opposed to transient homelessness, as he has been unhoused for greater than one year.[6] This patient has all the possible obstacles to obtaining long-term safe housing. He has a severe and persistent mental illness for which he does not take medication and may be treatment-refractory, he abuses drugs and alcohol and is repeatedly incarcerated, he is rumored to have a history of a sex offense (registered sex offenders may have severe limitations on where they can live for legal reasons, but those with reports of sexual violence in their past are also difficult to place), and he becomes violent when intoxicated and psychotic. It is also likely, given his chronic history of drugs and mental illness, that he has experienced early-onset cognitive impairment.

There are overt and covert reasons that homeless patients end up in the ED. In the second case, the overt or stated reason for removal by police was the patient's belligerent behavior and concern for his poor self-care. The more covert reasons probably have to do with the frustration of the officers who deal with him on a daily basis, the pressure on social service agencies to keep their clients out of the public eye, and the varying tolerance level of passersby in the station of this kind of behavior. In the short term, admitting him involuntarily to the hospital will provide him with a safe, warm, and dry place to stay; nutritious meals; clean clothes; and psychotropic medication to treat his symptoms, as well as a safe detoxification from alcohol and other drugs. In the time he is in the hospital it is hoped that he will not attack anyone, not get arrested, and can possibly gain insight into his situation and be more accepting of help. Hospitalization, however, will also deprive him of his liberty, forcing him in most hospital settings to stay inside 24 hours per day. Without appropriate supports in the community—and perhaps even despite them—he is likely to relapse soon after discharge. Hospitalization may or may not lead to safe and appropriate long-term housing. In cities that utilize a Housing First model, patients who are chronically homeless may be eligible to have housing placement expedited as a way of reducing service utilization and saving money overall, as opposed to requiring patients to be "housing ready" by meeting a series of criteria for being in treatment or seeking employment. Placement in stable and appropriate housing with community supports has been shown to reduce hospitalization; however, resources are scarce.[8]

There is certainly a fatigue that can develop from repeated visits from patients who seem to defy all attempts at providing mental health treatment and who return repeatedly to the ED year after year with the same issues, many of which may seem to derive from their lack of a stable and private place to live. These same patients frequently cycle in and out of correctional settings as well.[8] In terms of evidence-based attempts to break the cycle of homelessness in the mentally ill, the Critical Time Intervention model of case management works on the premise that providing intensive case management services after release to the community can prevent homelessness and re-hospitalization and could be applicable to this patient's situation.[9] However, he would have to be willing to accept that intervention.

The third case raises many issues that need to be considered when evaluating patients who are homeless with children. It seems reasonable that the woman described has experienced a series of overwhelming stressors that are leading to her anxiety, crying spells, and difficulty coping. Homelessness is obviously stressful for children and families and can have long-term consequences for children, including interfering with continuation of education, disruption of family and social networks, and exposure to violence.[10] A well-meaning caseworker, seeing a woman who is unable to calm down, asks the question that she is taught to ask: are you suicidal? Unable to "contract for safety," the patient is sent to the ED to assess her risk of harm to herself and her children. This is a case that poignantly exhibits the limitations of the hospital or crisis center to address this woman's issues, which are quite concrete: she needs financial help to get back on her feet and provide for her family; she needs assistance with finding safe, affordable housing and support through a difficult time, including grieving the departure of her spouse. Even if there are resources to set her up with mental health treatment, there remains the problem of how she is going to find a job, new housing, and essentially start over. She likely fears that if she is labeled as having a psychiatric illness, she may risk losing her children. Providing education and enlisting support can sometimes be the most helpful intervention for a homeless patient in distress, as well as supporting the patient through the process of navigating social services agencies. Peer advocate support might also be an option if available. Mental health treatment is likely to be a supportive treatment focused on goal-setting and problem-solving, at least in the short term.

In summary, asking very simple questions about where patients live and if they have a stable and permanent home can open a door to a more thorough understanding of what they are struggling with and how to provide an appropriate disposition. The informed clinician who is familiar with local services and resources will be better able to provide care in the ED setting.

Key Clinical Points

- Assessing housing status should be included in any comprehensive ED psychiatric evaluation, as it provides crucial information about the patient's daily context and informs treatment planning and disposition.
- Mental health treatment is of limited efficacy when concrete needs are not also addressed. Psychiatrists who work in ED or crisis center settings should have a familiarity with the social service resources in their community, even if they are not responsible for providing direct referrals.
- Chronic homelessness is associated with comorbidity of mental illness, substance abuse, forensic history, and history of trauma.
- Homeless families face unique challenges in maintaining a stable environment for their children, as they may also be uprooted from social networks.

REFERENCES

1. National Coalition for the Homeless fact sheet: Who is homeless? 2009; accessed online 11/7/2014, http://www.nationalhomeless.org/factsheets/who.html
2. New York City Coalition for the Homeless: Basic facts about homelessness in New York; accessed online 11/7/2014, http://www.coalitionforthehomeless.org/the-catastrophe-of-homelessness/facts-about-homelessness/
3. Montauk SL. The homeless in America: Adapting your practice. *American Family Physician.* 2006;74:1132–1138.
4. Zorza, J. Woman battering: A major cause of homelessness. *Clearinghouse Review* 1991; 25(4). Qtd. in National Coalition Against Domestic Violence, The importance of financial literacy, Oct. 2001.
5. Current Statistics on the Prevalence and Characteristics of People Experiencing Homelessness in the United States. Accessed 11/17/14 at ww.samhsa.gov
6. Henry M, Cortes A, Morris S. The 2013 Annual Homeless Assessment Report (AHAR) to Congress. Accessed online 11/17/14 at https://www.hudexchange.info/resources/documents/AHAR-2013-Part1.pdf
7. US Department of Housing and Urban Development Office of Policy Development and Research. The applicability of housing first models to persons with serious mental illness. July 2007. Accessed online 11/7/2014 at http://www.huduser.org/portal/publications/hsgfirst.pdf
8. Lamb HR, Weintraub L. Persons with severe mental illness in jails and prisons: A review. *Psychiatric Services.* 1998;49(4):483–492 (suppl).
9. Herman C, Conover S, Felix A et al. Critical time intervention, an empirically supported model for preventing homelessness in high risk groups. The Journal of Primary Prevention. Published online June 2007.
10. Kilmer R, Cook, R, Crusto C, et al. Understanding the ecology and development of children and families experiencing homelessness: Implications for

practice, supportive services and policy. American Journal of Orthopsychiatry 2012, 82(3): 389–401 DOI: 10.1111/j.1939-0025.2012.01160.x 389

FURTHER READING

McQuiston, HL. "Homelessness and Behavioral Health in the New Century" and "The Role of Psychiatry in Permanent Supported Housing." In: McQuiston HL, Sowers W, Ranz JM, Feldman JM, eds. *Handbook of Community Psychiatry.* New York: Springer;2012 (supplemental).